PSYCHOANALYSIS
AND
EATING DISORDERS

Edited by
Jules R. Bemporad, M.D.
David B. Herzog, M.D.

© 1989 The American Academy of Psychoanalysis
Published by The Guilford Press
A Division of Guilford Publications
72 Spring Street, New York, NY 10012

This volume was published simultaneously as *The Journal of the
American Academy of Psychoanalysis*, Volume 17, Number 1, Spring 1989.

ISBN 0-89862-388-X

Last digit is print number: 9   8   7   6   5   4   3   2   1

Printed in the United States of America

PSYCHOANALYSIS AND EATING DISORDERS

Guest Editors
Jules R. Bemporad, M.D.
David B. Herzog, M.D.

Contents

INTRODUCTION

Once considered quite rare, eating disorders are now encountered with increasing frequency by most clinicians. These forms of psychopathology have become so commonplace as to merit extensive coverage in the lay press. Equal attention has come from professional groups so that, in addition to a wealth of articles and books, there is even a separate journal dedicated to the investigation of eating disorders. Yet, in spite of being widely studied, eating disorders remain poorly understood, with disputes revolving around their diagnosis, etiology, and appropriate treatment.

Psychoanalysis had been aware of anorexia nervosa well before this disorder became fashionable. As early as 1889, Freud wrote to Fleiss that "the well known anorexia nervosa of girls seems to be . . . to be a melancholia occurring where sexuality is undeveloped. Loss of appetite—in sexual terms, loss of libido (Freud, 1889/ 1954). In the ensuing years, this disorder has been reinterpreted along the lines of each new development in psychoanalytic thought, so that to trace the history of its explanatory literature is almost to follow the historical course of psychoanalysis itself. Early traditional theories stressed that anorexia was a defense against wishes or fears of oral impregnation. Ego psychology focused on the weakness and ineffectiveness of the anorexic's ability to achieve individuation or self-reliance in adolescence, possibly as a result of disturbed early mother–child interactions. Adherents of an object-relations approach conceived of the disorder as the weakened psychological self's paranoid reaction against a powerful bad object which had become equated with the corporeal self. Family and interactional theorists commented on the family's exploitation of the anorexic child in order to maintain a pathological equilibrium within the home. Most recently, anorexia has been studied from the framework of self psychology, identifying failures in empathic mirroring and idealization during childhood.

As these formulations of anorexia nervosa were being delineated, a growing number of anorexics began presenting with episodes of bulimia, complicating the clinical and theoretical aspects of the illness. Finally, pure bulimia, without anorexia or hyperactivity, but with persistent self-induced emesis or laxative use, came to greater and greater attention of practitioners. These latter disorders appeared quite different, in terms of personality characteristics, psychodynamics, and past history, from the typical patient with "restrictive" anorexia nervosa. All the while, cultural standards for a feminine ideal were approaching, with mounting danger, sanctioned criteria not so disparate from clinical anorexia nervosa. It is difficult to determine how much of the "epidemic" of eating disorders that we are now witnessing is a result of the societal positing of thinness, self-control, and absolute autonomy as the epitome of successful femininity. One could also argue that the cultural condoning of anorexic behavior makes it harder to detect cases and, therefore, obscures an even-higher incidence of the disorder than reported in epidemiological surveys.

What is becoming clearer from the clinical experience of those who frequently treat eating-disordered patients is that this group of illnesses represents a varied and diverse group of individuals who defy easy generalization and may require a multimodal approach to treatment, tailored to each patient. It is also becoming frighteningly clear that these disorders carry a singularly poor prognosis with most forms of treatment. Garfinkel and Garner (1982) summarized the results of 25 recent follow-up studies on treated patients with anorexia nervosa. If a follow-up evaluation was performed at least a few years after the initial presentation and if patients of variable ages were seen, 30% were either dead as a result of the illness or chronically afflicted. The same authors also summarized follow-up studies that investigated general mental status in addition to symptoms of anorexia. A survey of these studies reveals that even in weight-recovered individuals, only 17–40% were symptom free: most continued to demonstrate significant depressive, obsessive–compulsive, or phobic symptoms.

Since bulimia nervosa was only classified as a distinct disorder in 1980 (DSM-III), to date, there are just a few published long-term studies. Although most short-term controlled trials of pharmacotherapy, cognitive–behavioral therapy, and group therapy have demonstrated marked symptomatic improvement, long-term studies have been less encouraging. A third to one-half of the patients were still ill at several years follow-up. In a recent prospective outcome study of outpatient bulimics seeking treatment at Massachusetts General Hospital, one-third were still in their index episode 35–42 months after evaluation. Of those who did recover (were asymptomatic for eight consecutive weeks) at some point during the follow-up, the great majority had at least one relapse. Notably, many of the "recovered" patients were compulsively exercising or eating restrictive diets, and depressive symptomatology was frequent.

It may be of particular relevance to psychoanalysts that Garfinkel and Garner conclude their review of prognosis with a favorable expectation from long-term therapies, which go beyond immediate symptom relief to modifying etiological factors, in the amelioration of the all-too-often negative outcome.

This special issue of the *Journal* hopes to share the clinical expertise of practitioners and researchers who daily treat and study individuals with eating disorders. The idea for a special issue grew out of a well-attended and well-received panel presented in Montreal in 1988. In addition to the four papers presented, other contributions were requested in order to capture the full variety of types of patients and issues that arise in the treatment of eating-disordered individuals. The contributors are all recognized as having made significant contributions to the treatment and understanding of these enigmatic yet most important group of disorders.

Jules R. Bemporad, M.D.
David B. Herzog, M.D.

References

Freud, S. (1889), *The Origins of Psychoanalysis*, Basic Books, New York, 1954.

Garfinkel, P. E., and Garner, D. M. (1982), *Anorexia Nervosa: A Multidimensional Perspective*, Brunner/Mazel, New York.

SELF PSYCHOLOGICAL REFLECTIONS ON THE ORIGINS OF EATING DISORDERS

RICHARD A. GEIST, Ed.D.

It is the intent of this paper to understand eating disorders as one major form of self pathology in which there has been both a "traumatic" and chronic disturbance in the empathic connectedness between parents and child. I will offer the hypothesis that what we see clinically as anorexia and bulimia represent two variations of a defensive structure mobilized to cope with a specific, sudden, and prolonged disruption in the early parent–child relationship (or more accurately, the archaic self–selfobject dimension of the parent–child relationship). Such a massive failure, through its particular disruption of the empathic milieu that maintains the integrity of the child's self, prevents the internalization of certain soothing and tension-regulating structures. It promotes dissociative defenses that become congruent with the more chronic empathic failures that exist (Geist, 1984), although in disparate form, in the families of both anorectic and bulimic women. The interweaving of these acute and cumulative developmental empathic failures (and the resulting structural deficits) becomes the childhood anlage of eating disorders; the primordial foundation for the adolescent's later attempt to fill in the structural deficit (to substitute for the frustrated selfobject needs) by symbolically recreating within the symptoms of anorexia and bulimia both the danger to the self and the efforts at self restoration.

Such a hypotheses, derived from the author's individual long-term psychotherapy with 20 eating-disorder patients,* represents an attempt to begin to determine the relationship between the general features of self pathology and the specific characteristics of a given clinical symptom. For it is only as the specific deficits that exist in the psyche of eating-disorder patients are mapped out as a clinical entity that it will be possible to determine and "spell

Richard A. Geist is a Clinical Associate, Department of Psychiatry, Massachusetts General Hospital, and Clinical Instructor, Harvard Medical School.

*All patients were females between the ages of 14 and 40. They were seen between 1 and 4 times per week for between 2 and 10 years.

out more specifically how the degree, timing, and combination of the various selfobject failures created these particular structural deficit and no others" (A. Ornstein, personal communication).

During the past few years several reports have emerged within the psychoanalytic literature that support the notion that early developmental deficits contribute significantly to the origin of eating disorders. Brenner (1983) stressed the failure of these patients to have internalized sufficient maternal functions. Goodsitt (1983) conceptualized eating disorders as involving a deficit in self regulating functions. Casper (1981) viewed bulimic symptomatology as an abortive effort to consolidate a defective self. Sugarman and Kurash (1982), relying on the theoretical formulations of Mahler, posited a core developmental failure for bulimic patients occurring at the practicing subphase of separation–individuation, a defect that interferes with the girl's capacity to evoke self and object representations. Lerner (1983) utilized case material to emphasize a developmentally impaired capacity to symbolize because of failure of attunement of the mother in the early parent–child relationship. Swift and Letven (1984), attempting a psychoanalytic formulation based on the work of Balint and Kohut, suggested that these patients demonstrated a "basic fault" in their ego structure, specifically "an impairment in certain ego functions which regulate tension" (p. 489). Finally, Bruch (1985), in attempting to summarize her life-long contribution to the field, emphasized that continuing paucity of parental responses to "child initiated clues appeared to be related to the patients' deficits in self-concept and in hunger awareness" (p. 17). She concludes by suggesting that her ideas have a close resemblance to those expressed by Kohut in his psychology of the self.

In mentioning these works, it seems important to recognize that there is growing agreement among researchers representing disparate psychoanalytic vantage points that early developmental deficits play a significant role in the etiology of eating disorders. It is the purpose of this paper to investigate these deficits from a self psychological perspective. Information obtained in this way, from an empathic merger with patients over time, is experience-near data — very different and often diametrically opposed to that acquired through structured interviews, psychological tests, and behavioral rating scales. Experience-near data is collected by feeling and thinking our way into the patient's psychic reality and understanding her world from her personal biased perspective. By pursuing this line of thought, however, I am in no way suggesting that the resulting developmental picture is an objective rendering of actual happenings; rather, my purpose is to report how eating-disorder patients experienced certain aspects of their growing up. Thus I am shifting our perspective from an interest in the objective etiology of eating disorders *qua* illness to an interest in the subjective, genetic matrix from which these patients experience their eating disorders as having arisen.

EMPATHY AND THE DEVELOPMENT OF THE SELF

The human self, experienced as a sense of wholeness, aliveness, and vigor, an independent center of initiative over time and through space, is the essence of one's psychological being (Tolpin, 1980); but its very developmental life is linked with an element it cannot realistically control. Only a responsive selfobject milieu can provide those experiences of living that facilitate the transformation of the infant's potential into a creative aliveness and realness — a self structure with joyful interests and self affirming initiative. This human caretaking environment, because it provides those confirming, calming, and sustaining functions — mirroring, idealizing, and partnering — that have yet to be internalized by the child, is experienced as part of the self. In the language of self psychology, we refer to the empathic responses from such an environment — to those perceived aspects of another that shore up the self — as selfobject functions. Empathically informed parental selfobject responses constitute the external precursors — the "provisional psychic structure" — that contribute to and foster the internal psychic structures of the self.

It is in the reciprocal world of the subjectively experienced self-selfobject tie that empathy assumes its central position. For empathy, here defined as the capacity to place oneself inside another's psychic reality and experience the world from that person's subjective vantage point, informs the parents of the child's needs. The clinical sense of the word defines how parents (and therapists) collect the data with which to understand their children (and patients). Empathy, of course, can be correct or incorrect; but where parental empathy is accurate, the child will feel understood on what can only be described as a core level of her being. Beyond its use as a methodological tool for collecting data, then, empathy becomes a psychological holding environment that silently facilitates development. While a thorough evaluation of the developmentally mutative aspects of empathy are beyond the purview of the present paper, it is my belief that when accurately understood in her subjective way of viewing the world, the child experiences a number of important self enhancing consequences that reverberate, however disparately, throughout each state of development. And *pari passu*, when traumatic empathic failure occurs, there may temporarily be a total collapse of selfobject responsiveness, requiring emergency measures to maintain the integrity of the self. Because I shall postulate a major disruption in the empathic milieu of all eating-disorder patients, it seems important to outline several self enhancing qualities of such an empathic environment in childhood.*

First, when a child feels understood, she experiences a sense of realness — an awareness of being alive, personally present, and invested in one's own functioning, activities, and capacities. Empathy, by its mere existence, becomes the sustenance that, as Kohut (1980) suggests, keeps the self psychologically alive. Just as oxygen maintains the integrity of the physical self, so empathy bathes the psychological self in the nutriment that guarantees its survival. Empathy thus remains an important guardian of the individual's narcissistic equilibrium throughout life.

Second, when a child feels understood, empathy fosters the integration of new experiences. In the context of another's understanding presence, both external and internal experiences can be contained. Through such containment, an individual can develop a wider experiencing self with the potential for inclusion and modulation of an increasing variety of affects, feelings, thoughts, wishes, and fantasies. When such understanding exists, the individual can tolerate holding certain feelings that her ego does not yet have the capacity to actualize and master.

Third, when an individual feels understood, empathy fosters an important quality of communication. For, the very fact of having been understood is tantamount to a validation of successfully hav-

---

*In the clinical setting, empathy is a methodological tool that defines how the self psychologist collects his data. On another level, however, empathy transcends its use as a methodological tool and becomes a psychological holding environment that silently facilitates development. As Goldberg (1983) states, "The most promising field for a future classification of empathy would seem to be its consideration along developmental lines which would most cogently account for the therapeutic benefit of its employment" (p. 168). The present section is merely an attempt to begin to outline such developmental possibilities.

ing communicated how one feels. The gratification and satisfaction inherent in being known by another fosters progressively higher levels of "empathic resonance" (Kohut, 1984; Wolf, 1983) between two people as understanding begins to replace the actual gratification of archaic selfobject needs. Such resonance creates one of the most powerful bonds that can exist between human beings.

Fourth, the feeling of being understood allows the child a healthy sense of having created an omnipotent selfobject, which, in turn, confirms the perfection of the self. As this sense of omnipotence is sustained by an understanding milieu, empathy fosters not only the slow disillusionment of omnipotence (via transmuting internalization of psychic structure), but also the continuation of omnipotence in the form of the capacity to create; to play symbolically with fanciful ideas and feelings over which one has absolute control. Thus empathy becomes the guardian of creative potentiality.

Finally, when a child feels understood, empathy allows for the actual experiencing of selfobject failure. In other words, in every child–parent relationship, just as in every patient–therapist relationship, selfobject failure will occur. Neither parents nor therapists can maintain perfect empathic responsiveness; but whether the child can utilize these optimal failures in the service of taking over parental functions (thus building self structure) or whether the feelings of emptiness, loss, disappointment, and lowered self-esteem become split off and/or repressed is contingent on their occurring in an ongoing psychological climate of empathy. As Tolpin (1983) suggests,

> When parents in the role of selfobjects constitute an expectable psychological environment, the child who flops and fails is put to rights . . . the child mentally holds onto an impersonalized, transformed intrapsychic replica of the supportive verbal and nonverbal exchanges after the fall. These intrapsychic replicas (structures and functions) are built up into the child's own capacities and these help the child to recover his or her emotional balance and to stand firm again. (p. 368)

What is important to reiterate here is that these "corrective developmental dialogues" leading to transmuting internalizations can only take place if the individual child first actually experiences the failures. Such feelings, however, can only be experienced in a reliable empathic environment.

In sum, empathy allows a world of shared meanings where one's aliveness and realness become actual. Without empathy, this shared space between individuals becomes empty space, the presence of nothingness; the tendrils of the self begin to wither and to be replaced by defensive structures that protect its incipient integrity and cohesiveness.

This brief comment on empathy's role in the evolution and maintenance of the self leads directly to a description of the initial traumatic empathic failure that contributes to the development of anorexia nervosa and bulimia. Such a traumatic insult to the self leads to a fear of psychic emptiness, loss of creative living, and fragmentation, resulting in psychological depletion, loss of vitality, and threats to self cohesion.

THE INITIAL TRAUMA

Eating-disorder patients lack the empathic resonance that results from the psychological connectedness inherent in an archaic self–selfobject tie. Rather, they "remember"—through the controlled regression made possible by intensive psychotherapy—a disturbance in the empathic connectedness with parents, which occurs between 18 and 36 months when the self is in its more formidable stages of development. Although we call this disturbance a "trauma" from our experience-distant perspective, the patient does not experience "trauma" in the usual sense of a potentially rememberable event, which, under the proper therapeutic circumstances, can later be reported with vivid recall. Rather, these patients have experienced, as Winnicott (1974) aptly suggests in another context, "nothing happening when something might profitably have happened" (p. 106).

I was first alerted to such an experience of emptiness or nothingness through its recreation in the transference in the form of a complaint that "nothing is happening" in the therapy. In other words, as selfobject needs became remobilized in the treatment, each of my patients began to experience me as potentially able to provide them with an unknown something that I failed to proffer. Intense frustration ensued and the patients' capacity for communicating within the therapeutic space, particularly via free association, diminished. However, when their insistent demands were recognized, not as resistance or entitlement that they had to overcome or grow out of, but as rightful attempts to recreate in the therapy a feeling that was never entirely experienced, I generally witnessed a strengthening of the self that allowed the emergence of subjective memories highlighting an early disturbance in the empathic connectedness to parents. As will be apparent in the following two examples, such memories illustrate the contextual meaning of "trauma." Each report occurs following the experiencing of emptiness within the transference.

Case 1: Jennifer

Jennifer, a 21-year-old single woman, came to her therapy hour excited. She hadn't vomited in a month and that was the first time that had happened in 5 years. (I acknowledged her excitement.) She then said that she had been feeling sad, but wasn't sure what about. (I wondered whether the excitement of her binging and vomiting had perhaps been regulating certain feelings until now.) Jennifer said she thought that was true because she was feeling more of everything since not vomiting. There was a silence and then she went on to tell me about a friend of her mother who had died recently. "I feel sad; it was so sudden. I'm not only sad, I'm scared. If I don't vomit, there'll be nothingness. It's so scary to experience nothingness; that's what's unbearable. I first began vomiting when my boy friend broke up with me. I guess he was sort of a sustaining person for me. I guess it prevented me from feeling when he left too. My mother wants to take me shopping. I'm worried about how it will go. She's so intrusive." She then reported a long history of enemas and maternal preoccupation with her bowel movements, and said, "my mother want to knit me a scarf and even that's too intrusive. I'm worried that she'll disappoint me when we go shopping and that I'll vomit again." (I wondered if she meant she'd vomit as a way to deal with the emptiness resulting from the loss of connectedness with her.) Jennifer replied, "Yes, it doesn't matter where it comes in and goes out. (I said, "You mean doing to yourself what she did to you with the enemas.") "Yes, it's not so different from the enemas." A long silence ensues. Then she asks, "But what about the emptiness, my terrible fear of it?" (I knew enough about her history at this point to say that I had a feeling that it had already happened, that she had been connected to her mother and then suddenly there was nothingness, and that somehow there must have been no sustaining person to help her deal with it when she was little. I started to say more but she interrupted me, crying at this point.) "You're right. I remember. I only have vague memories. My mother's mother dying when I was just under two. There was nothingness. I remember the nothingness and this may sound strange, but after that nothingness the only thing I remember was waking up on the toilet. My mother's focus was all on my bowels. (I said, "As if the focus on your bowels, one isolated part of you instead of all your creative productions, stimulated you and your mother out of the nothingness.") "Yeah, and then when my next sibling was born things were better; they talked of him as filling the gap. Everyone was all excited again and I joined with them in it; only as I look back on it I don't know how real it was. I wouldn't know it wasn't real without me feeling real now. In fact my eating wasn't real; it didn't have any pleasure in it."

Case 2: Stephanie

Stephanie, an 18-year-old college freshman, began the session with the following: "I hate going into the cafeteria because everyone watches me. I hate being watched." (I asked what it felt like when she was watched.) "It's like everyone is saying, oh, she's eating, so if she can eat, she doesn't have any problems." ("So you're afraid of being watched because people won't see the whole of you, just the fragment of your eating and then misunderstand your needs.") "Exactly," she said. A short silence followed while she sat back in her chair and took off her coat. "I've been misunderstood an awful long time. Even in my last therapy. The psychologist said, okay, we'll take two interviews to diagnose the problem and then find a solution. The problem was decision making and we worked on making decisions. How can anyone make a diagnosis in two sessions and how can I work with decision making until I know how I feel about it? It's like eating. It's like a friend sent me an article on anorexia; the experts were quoted. How did she know it would apply to me? It gets me so aggravated." ("More examples of your feeling misunderstood, specifically of people watching the outside of you and ignoring your inner feelings.") "All this goes back so far." Here she becomes very sad and teary, and after a short silence asks, "What do you think it's like to be insane?" (I suggested perhaps it was like trying to deal with unbearable agonies.) "All those people locked up for years, since they were so young. It feels like it could go back to when they were two or three. No one to help them. I'd rather be dead than know my self is not all there, that's what's so unbearable, knowing my self is not there, nothing happening inside of me." (I said, "Yes, the deadness is a way of coping with the agony of the break up of your self when you were very young.") "Maybe if someone had known they could have helped." (I agreed that some one could help.) She then asked, "What am I going to do about my eating?" (I told her that the very fact she was able to ask me was a hopeful sign, because she was bringing into the therapy the right of every child to borrow an adult's strength when they were in difficulty and it was her capacity to borrow my strength and mine to allow it that would lead to a solution.)

Within the vacuity of these patients' memories, the experience of nothingness reflects not so much the loss of specific parental selfobject functions (although, this does in fact occur), but rather the more total loss of the psychological oxygen that keeps the self alive. (Total refers to a period beyond which the child cannot maintain the cohesiveness of the self.) Such nothingness appears to be different from the "aloneness" that Adler and Buie (1979) describe so eloquently in the borderline patient. For most women with eating disorders do not experience the same conviction that there is no one in reality who is really there for them. They do not lack the capacity to summon a fantasy of a positive, sustaining relationship; nor do they, with the same consistency, have frightening or negative images or fantasies of important people. In their regressive states, eating-disorder patients do not experience a loss of contact with reality in general; they experience disintegration anxiety, "the threatened loss of self cohesion maintaining responses of the empathic selfobject" (Kohut, 1984, p. 19). The emptiness of eating-disorder patients reflects more the quality of a depleted and dying self in the context of the dessication of its sustaining ambience. They experience a withering of that creative living where feelings, moods, and events can be communicated or symbolically represented, played with, and actualized; and they begin to lose both the capacity to comprehend what they are experiencing and to integrate it into an aspect of a more completely experiencing self.

Such a trauma seems to occur during a specific developmental period, and while a full discussion of this period is beyond the scope of this paper, it is important to recall, from a self psychological vantage point, several developmental phenomena that are in process at the time of the trauma. (For, as Kohut (1984) has suggested, our experience-distant theories of normality do influence our responses to experience-near data.)

1. The self structure has attained its initial and tentative cohesiveness, but remains quite vulnerable to empathic failures.
2. The child, via attempts at bodily mastery—toilet training, walking unself-consciously, speaking in sentences—holds up her creative, productive self to be admired, confirmed, and validated. This process, when mirrored with pride by the parents, facilitates the joy and excitement of this age group and helps the child's archaic grandiosity to become more integrated.
3. The child begins to attain the capacity for symbol formation and self reflection, making it possible for the use of fantasy and play to ease the slow disillusionment of the child's omnipotent control over the selfobject.
4. The child's affects, those "somatic responses to stimulation of the nervous system," in the context of an empathic milieu, have the potential during this stage for becoming feeling. As Basch (1983) puts it, "the conscious awareness of an affective event as a subjective experience which we call feeling, becomes a possibility" (p. 117).
5. The child's tentatively cohesive self begins to strengthen its boundaries by relying on its selfobjects, not only for echoing and confirming responses, but as a selfobject "antagonist against whom self assertion mobilizes healthy aggression which promotes the cohesive strength of the self" (Wolf, 1980, p. 126).

It is not surprising in this context that what we discern later in the symptomatology of eating disorders reflects the derailment of developmental tasks of this age group. This symptomatology includes a fragmentation-prone self experienced as feelings of incompetence, inadequacy, and phoniness; a self whose split-off grandiosity is not available to contribute to self-esteem and occasionally overwhelms the patient's ego with intense shame; a self deprived of any extensive use of fantasy and unself-conscious play; a self that is in touch with affect, but has little access to feeling states; and a self whose healthy self assertion has broken down into quietly simmering narcissistic rage, which is expressed in the form of perfection (Geist, 1984).

As empathy, the psychological nutriment for the self, atrophies, the child has no context in which to experience her feeling of emptiness and is thus deprived of the potential for internalizing parental selfobject functions. Instead, the self, lacking the sustaining selfobject tie, begins to lose its feeling of aliveness, has no way to modulate the intense affective state, feels increasingly misunderstood and unable to borrow the strength of the parents. As the child then searches for emergency measures to protect the depleted self, emptiness becomes split off, a dissociated element that begins to function separately from the rest of the personality. Both Jennifer and Stephanie were aware, for example, that they continued to exist, to play, and to eat, but, as Jennifer recognized retrospectively, it was a mechanical, self-conscious kind of eating devoid of any pleasure and spontaneity. In this dissociated state, food can be accepted as medicine, or eating habits can be altered through various short-term behavioral manipulations, but the creative enjoyment of food can never become a pleasurable integrated, unself-conscious function. For the split-off emptiness must be reexperienced and reintegrated into a more consolidated self before true filling up is possible.

Stephanie offered a vivid illustration of this dissociated state a few months after the interview I reported. As the idealized relationship with the therapist became safe enough to allow the experiencing of earlier feelings, she began to reexperience in the treatment the split-off emptiness. Reintegration made possible by the selfobject transference (increasing consolidation of the self) allowed increasing depressive states to be modulated. During that time Stephanie went home for a weekend. Afterwards she described it to me. "Before I went away I had my first good meal in years. I mean I enjoyed it and didn't think about what or how much I was taking in. I just ate normally. I felt different, more like me. When I got home, I continued to eat that way and I found myself looking back at picture albums from when I was between one and five. I had never noticed before how strange that little girl looked. She wasn't me. There were pictures of her. She was eating and playing, but it wasn't part of her. You could see on her face that it was false; I mean, no one else could, but suddenly I could. I never really could play, but I never knew I couldn't." I acknowledged the increasing vitality of her self and the resulting capacity to recognize her earlier state. She replied, "What made me notice was the contrast between how I felt eating now and how I know she ate and lived. But before I got in touch with this emptiness, I never knew it was strange to be like her."

Winnicott (1974) has stated,

> The basis of all learning (as well as of eating) is emptiness. . . . But if emptiness was not experienced at the beginning, then it turns up as a state

that is feared, yet compulsively sought after. . . . In some patients emptiness needs to be experienced, and this emptiness belongs to the past, to the time before the degree of maturity had made it possible for emptiness to be experienced. (p. 107)

In self psychological terms it can be said that the basis for all eating is in the experience of nontraumatic optimal failure, minor failures that, as parents help their children to experience and integrate, foster the internalization of new functions, and enable children to experience the feeling of emptiness. When the selfobject milieu breaks down traumatically, however, the patient must find ways to fill in the resulting structural deficits as best she can.

Eating-disorder patients' attempts to fill in the self's structural deficits include a wide range of behavioral phenomena; frantic business, sexualization of isolated drives, overstimulating physical activities, petty thefts, a hyperinvestment in the intellectual aspects of communication, and compliance are some of the more common strategies. Although disparate in their outward appearance, these behavioral and psychological activities are attempts to preserve that sector of the self that has been at least precariously established "despite the serious insufficiencies in the development-enhancing matrix of the selfobjects of childhood" (Kohut, 1984, p. 115). For example, Jennifer described the sexualization of an isolated drive when she stated that the only thing she remembered after the nothingness was waking up on the toilet. Here she speaks for all those bulimic patients I have seen in long-term psychotherapy. Each one has experienced—previous to the onset of symptoms—the prolonged sexualization of anal aspects of themselves as a strategy to preserve one small component of their creative, productive self during the 18–36 month period of growth. Such a focus on anality has nothing to do with sexuality as a primary drive. It occurs in reaction to a failure of the parental selfobject at a time that corresponds to toilet training, a failure of the selfobject to appreciate the child's total creative productions. As a reaction, the child, instead of using this developmental period to make important contributions to the consolidation and enrichment of her self, uses a sexualization of one component part, bowel functioning, to ward off serious forms of depletion and emptiness.

To illustrate each of the abovementioned attempts to preserve the vulnerable self structure would take us beyond the scope of this paper. What remains important, however, is to understand the healthy motivation contained in such activities so that we do not *ipso facto* curtail self preserving behavior under the misguided assumption that we are providing ego controls with which the patient will then identify. Thus when a patient suddenly increases her exercise regime in the hospital setting, her behavior should act as a signal for the staff to search out their own selfobject failures rather than punish the patient via restrictions and other forms of punitive limit setting. Obviously one is guided by the medical needs of an individual patient, but it has been my experience that only when such activities are understood as healthy attempts to shore up the self in the face of selfobject failure can the patient feel understood enough to remobilize her early selfobject needs within the treatment and thus reopen the door to building compensatory structures via the process of transmuting internalization.

It is also important to remember that attempts to fill in the structural deficits of the self seem to be influenced by and occur within the context of the more chronic empathic failures that eating-disorder patients remember from their childhood. In a earlier paper (Geist, 1984), I have delineated these failures and their implications for a specific self psychological therapeutic approach; here I will merely summarize those themes that seem to have defined the patient's selfobject ambience previous to the onset of her eating disorder.

Shattered Sense of Wholeness

The eating-disorder patient experiences herself as having lived in a milieu permeated by repeated parental misunderstanding of her need to be perceived as a whole person. Patients report a long history of fragmentation-producing responses. These responses include overattention to bodily appearances with total or partial disregard of inner feelings; scrutiny of momentary behaviors, but a denial of their temporal or spacial relativity; and preoccupation with negative aspects of their performance while denying the joy and pride inherent in the total production. In other words, when the eating-disorder patient peered into the mirror of the parents, she perceived not the sustaining reflection of her whole body self, but a prismatic image of isolated parts. As one patient poignantly suggested,

It was as though I never got *me* back from anyone in my family; instead I got back the parts of me that were wrong or bad. It made me feel crazy. When that happened, I would look into five different mirrors in my house and I always saw something different. It was like listening to a tape; you sound different than you sound to yourself. Who I was got all confused and I felt totally lost. No one could see it then, but it made me feel like my head and my stomach weren't connected.

Eating-disorder patients experienced themselves as living in a world where they were continually defined by what others perceived as the negative particle of their more complete being.

The Subordination of Mirroring to Defensive Identification

The eating-disorder patient experienced herself as having possessed an exquisite sensitivity to the unspoken needs and wishes of her mother. Having partially failed to internalize parental selfobject functions (and thus having failed to develop a cohesive self), her tuning into and fitting into the internal state of the parent appears to have represented a defensive attempt to preserve her connectedness to her mother. The child experienced herself as taking in characteristics of the mother that remained untransmuted, in other words, aspects of the mother that the patient knew the mother perceived as special, but that the patient did not feel belonged to her (the patient's) self. Within this collusive bond, compliance fostered subordination of the child's self to the subservient position of a narcissistic extension of the mother. As one patient recalled,

it felt like I had no choice, either I had to believe or feel what she (mother) did or I lost her. I mean, I didn't feel she didn't love me; it was just that she was so hurt, like she felt she wasn't a good mother if we weren't the same. You know, she baked cookies and if I didn't like them, it was devastating to her. And I would lose her in some way I can't explain. But if I did say I liked them, I lost me. It got so I really didn't know if I liked them or not. I know it has something to do with me now. I'm terrified of being like her and just as scared of not being like her.

Thus the eating-disorder patient felt compelled to fit in with the mother's way of being in order to preserve the self–selfobject tie, but the compliant preservation of such a tie meant the vitiating of that internalization that would allow her to experience herself as a uniquely enduring and cohesive individual.

The Experiencing of Precocity

Eating-disorder patients report having grown up in where they frequently experienced themselves as the _____ adult. Such precocity, which included the premature development of social and intellectual skills, is also remembered as including a secretive, eroticized relationship with the father during the girl's oedipal years and thereafter. In the role of mother of the house these girls recall a special connectedness with father in two specific ways: (1) as a relationship in which both acknowledged, usually nonverbally, the father's preference for his daughter in the context of their unwitting exclusion of the mother; and (2) as a relationship in which the girl experienced a basic feeling of her father's sustaining presence. As one patient reported,

> When I think back, I can't remember her [the mother] as being in my life when I was little. I know she was physically there, but all my memories are with my father — sharing things like going to the science museum, eating a hamburg at Burger King, my building model ships while he built his model ships, being able to share a joke with him or an important conversation, sitting on his lap when I ate. I don't know what she did. Why do you think I can't remember her being there?

On the one hand, then, the father's fostering of a uniquely exclusive relationship with his daughter provided in an overstimulating manner (and in the service of his needs) that mirroring and echoing for which the girl yearned. Thus he contributed to his daughter's building of defensive structures, those structures that maintain the self but do not allow for any transmuting internalizations to occur. In his capacity as a sustaining presence, however, he helped her build compensatory structures. In other words, through the partnering she experienced with her father, she can, in fact, internalize a modicum of psychic structure. (As I have previously suggested, it has been my experience that when fathers are unable to accomplish this task, we see borderline rather than narcissistic pathology (Geist, 1984).)

The Lack of a Calming, Soothing Other

The retrospective perceptions of eating-disorder patients suggest a chronic dearth of available adults with whose admired source of soothing and comforting the child could merge when she needed a lift. Rather the patient remembers herself as the comforting,

GEIST

soothing, organizing force in the home. As one patient recalled, "My mother would always ask which dress she should wear, or whether she looked okay or whether her cooking was good. Even my father, although he did it less, would ask my advice about things I didn't know about. It felt as though I was being a mother to my parents so I couldn't use them for support." The acquisition of self soothing and tension modulating structures via transmuting internalization was partially thwarted; and it appears to be this structural deficit that contributes to the dearth of self regulating functions in eating, sleeping, exercising, and the like, that seems to exist in eating-disorder patients. In order to prevent the anxiety that arises in the wake of such deficiencies, these patients substitute a rote perfectionism for the self soothing so necessary for everyday life. The assumption that one's body self is perfect, that there is automatic self regulation and soothing, alleviates the anxiety that would occur upon discovering a perceived lack of control over her own functioning.

THE CHILDHOOD ANLAGE

The perception of an unempathic ambience of the family, combined with the initial trauma and self stimulating attempts to compensate for the missing structures of the self comprise the childhood anlage, the primoridal foundation for eating disorders. This anlage remains relatively encapsulated until adolescence when the teenage girl or young adult woman experiences for the second time a significant loss of a sustaining archaic selfobject milieu. This may take the form of the loss of a best friend, change of school, graduation, depression of a parent, or even a significant developmental achievement such as acceptance to college, in other words, a loss that, from our experience-distant perspective of normality, most adolescents can sustain. What makes such a loss different for the future eating-disorder patient is that, because of the failure to internalize sufficient psychic structure, there has not been a shift from the need for archaic self–selfobject support to higher levels of selfobject relationships. Most adolescents, for example, derive sustanence from knowing that they have the opportunity for belonging to groups that reflect their similar interests, values, and beliefs; they derive support from knowing there are admired adults whose strength they can borrow when in need of a lift; and they can rely on support from an atmosphere of friendly others who admire or at least appreciate their assets. Women with future eating disorders, while appearing to function in a similar manner to normal adolescents, do not experience themselves as existing in a milieu that resonates with the potential for empathic support. The loss of a best friend does not lead, after a period of sadness to the relatively confident expectation of finding others who can perform similar selfobject functions; rather the loss is experienced as a drying up of the archaic selfobject environment. For future eating-disorder patients, the adolescent's environmental surround remains the "external provisional psychic structure" that has yet to be transmuted into internal capacities. Any loss leaves the adolescent highly vulnerable to the reemergence of disintegrating anxiety and the accompanying fear of emptiness.

It is at this point that the patient once again "fears the awfulness of emptiness and in defense will organize a controlled emptiness by not eating . . . or else will ruthlessly fill up by a greediness which is compulsive and feels mad" (Winnicott, 1974, p. 107). Translated into self psychological terms, it is at this point that the adolescent fears the awfulness of disintegration anxiety and the accompanying feeling of emptiness. It is also at this point that the formerly used emergency measures—compliance, sexualization, stealing, exercising, and so forth, no longer are sufficient to preserve the remnants of the self. As Tolpin (1978) states,

When vigorous demands and appeals directed to the selfobjects are to no avail, disintegration anxiety and/or depletion anxiety ensues, and there is likely also to be a breakup of the child's healthy assertion into its disintegration product—narcissistic rage. The inner psychological states resulting from loss of cohesiveness (disintegration depletion, and/or narcissistic rage) can be manifested directly, can be given any kind of symbolic expression or representation, and can be sexualized. (p. 175)

Whereas before the onset of adolescence, the empty depletion is frequently sexualized or dealt with via those behavioral measures suggested above, the failure of these activities leads to its symbolic expression through the activity most closely related to emptiness— eating.* It has been my experience that in both anorexia and bu-

---

*Although beyond the scope of this paper, I have found that the fear of emptiness contributes to these patients' fear of being fat. If the acknowledgment of emptiness is necessary for filling up to take place, the fear of being fat becomes

limia, the controlled eating, binging, and vomiting contain, on a deep level, an attempt to recreate, within the symptoms, the archaic selfobject function that existed when mother and child were empathically connected. Thus, as the following example indicates, food and the related activities of eating, feeding, binging, and vomiting fill in the structural deficits in the self.

CAROL

Carol, a 24-year-old single woman, is a graduate student in English at a local university. She has been hospitalized for anorexia, but currently is not anorectic. During the course of treatment, bulimic symptoms have replaced the anorexia. At the time of this interview, however, she is beginning to relinquish these symptoms as well. Carol has been in treatment with me three times a week, for three years. I am her fourth therapist, although her current therapy is the only one she has sustained for more than a year.

She enters the office and sits for a moment, as is her custom. I typically wait for her to begin, although there are times when she still needs my help.

Carol: "Well, my parents came back last night from their European vacation. I went over to their house to say hello and decided to stay the night. It was okay seeing them. (As if this has been an aside, Carol then talks at length about how lonely she's been feeling lately, how none of her long-time friends seem to want to be with her any more. She assures me that the loneliness goes beyond her parents being away; she feels the loneliness has been growing for months now.)

"My emptiness must have something to do with the dream I had last night. I was on my way to my poetry class and was surrounded by a group of friends. They were talking to me, but I couldn't seem to relate to them. I wanted to, but just couldn't get outside of

---

tantamount to a fear of once again experiencing an overwhelming depletion. Similarly, the refusal to accept gifts, praise, and admiration protects one from ever having to acknowledge that one was "hungering" (i.e., empty) for such gratifications. It is the lack of self structure, however, that prevents the patient from modulating such feelings of emptiness and thus allowing the experience of nothing in tolerable doses.

myself to do it. It was strange, but during the dream I wet my bed. Do you think it's normal for a 24-year-old to wet her bed?"

Therapist: You mean you've had enough symptoms already and don't need another?"

Carol: That's exactly what I mean. I can't imagine having one more problem to worry about.

Therapist: Well, in answer to your question, it's unlikely that you'd develop a new and prolonged symptom at this point.

Carol: You know, none of my other therapists used to answer my questions. When you answer them, I can let myself feel real and go on; the answer isn't as important as the fact that you take them seriously. The wetting makes me think of my mother. She once told me that as a kid she and her two sisters were bedwetters. I used to be afraid to find out. When I was at boarding school as a teenager there were some girls who wet their beds, but I never gave it much thought.

Therapist: So you had her symptom just when she got back from her trip to Europe?

Carol: Yeah, it was their first night back, like I said. I stayed over and slept in my old bed. Oh, and when I woke up in the morning, I knew where I was. You know how I'm usually all disoriented when I wake up in my apartment. But I knew where I was, in fact, I said, "My mother gave me this bed." I sat up and said it out loud, almost as if it were still part of the dream.

Therapist: Almost as if you wet your mother, sort of searching for a comfortable lap to wet on?

Carol: I know that's right. When I woke up I felt cuddly and good and warm; it's been so long since I felt that way.

Therapist: And you weren't disoriented either, when you felt cuddly and warm.

Carol: I remember one other time in my life having a dream when I wet my bed, but I can't remember it.

(There was a five-minute silence.)

Carol: I was thinking about the people in the dream, how I'm changing and wondering if the friendships will continue.

Therapist: I know it's harder when two people have to change instead of just you.

Carol: Do you think I'll be able to make new friends if I lose them. I don't know if I could tolerate the emptiness. There were so many people in the dream. You know, one of the people was my old roommate from sophomore year at college, the one I confided in when I was first becoming anorectic. She was in this peer counseling program and she began trying to help me. We got real close, then when things really fell apart and I got hospitalized they wouldn't let her visit me and she just stayed away. When I got out at the end of the year, she had arranged for another roommate. I bumped into her every now and then, but wasn't the same. I think in the dream she was the one I wanted to be close to.

Therapist: You wanted to rejoin her after she dropped you — to get back to the sustaining feelings you had when you were first with her?

Carol: You think there was something good with my mother when I was real young, don't you?

Therapist: Yes, I do, then I think it got lost and for a long time you've been searching for a way to get back that something good, the good feelings you had about yourself when you felt connected with her.

Carol: My vomiting, it's like the wetting, isn't it? It's a way of finding her, isn't it?

Therapist: Yes, I think it is, sort of a way of creating what you need in the symptom; every little girl needs a shoulder that she can throw up on.

Carol: (Begins to cry) I know just when it was, at three years old, when we came back from California and she was sick for that year — that's from her — but I feel it right now. I know I lost her. It was like she sent me away, but I was still there. [She cries silently for the remainder of the hour.]

Therapist: I know we're right in the middle, but we do have to interrupt for now. [She continues to sit staring off into space.] It's particularly hard to be sent away today. (She gets up and leaves quietly.)

Andre Green (1973, quoted in Khan, 1978) has suggested that

One major capacity of the psychic structure is the capacity to cut off, to suspend an experience, white it is still going on. This is not for the purpose of observing the experience as in the conscious mental functioning, but to shut off the awareness of it in order to recreate it in one's own way later on.

For the eating-disorder patient, I am suggesting that it is the archaic self–selfobject tie that is being recreated in the extratherapeutic selfobject transference to food (i.e., early selfobject needs are remobilized in the hopes that food will supply the missing functions of the self). This conceptualization illuminates how when the adolescent once again fears the awfulness of self depletion and the accompanying feeling of emptiness, and her usual emergency measures fail to assure the self's survival, she symbolically recreates what she needs in that activity most closely related to emptiness, eating.

The subjectively experienced memories of these patients confirm that their mothers were highly preoccupied with food, eating, and cooking. It is not surprising, then, that these women, when confronting a second major selfobject failure, attempt to borrow their mothers' self regulating mechanisms—measures that appear far more reliable to the patient than the human selfobject. (It should be clear that the mother may not have been so unreliable throughout development, but that the incapacity of the patient to use her in the service of transmuting internalization leading to structure building predisposes the child to perceive her mother as continually unreliable.) Food, eating, and feeding activities thus become a reliable selfobject over which she has omnipotent control (with both the capacity to create and to destroy it).

Understanding food as an archaic selfobject further clarifies why it is used as a self regulating function, as defensive stimulation, and as protection against emptiness, why narcissistic rage is so intimately connected with the use of food, and ultimately, how food as archaic selfobject becomes reinvested with so much "primary childhood intensity" (Kohut, 1984), that giving up the symptom is a life or death issue. Consequently, the symptomatologies of anorexia and bulimia represent neither unconscious compromises, symbolically acted out control battles with parents, nor internalized societal preoccupation with thinness; rather, they actualize life and death struggles to maintain the integrity of the self and prevent disintegration anxiety.

References

Adler, G., and Buie, D. (1979), Aloneness and borderline psychopathology. *Int. J. Psycho-Anal., 60,* 83–96.
Basch, M. F. (1983), Empathic understanding: A review of the concept and some theoretical considerations. *J. Am. Psychoanal. Assoc., 31,* 101–125.

26 GEIST

Brenner, D. (1983), Self regulatory functions in bulimia. *Contemp. Psychother. Rev., 1*, 79-96.
Bruch, H. (1985), Four decades of eating disorders, in D. M. Garner and P. E. Garfinkel (Eds.), *Handbook of Psychotherapy for Anorexia Nervosa and Bulimia*, Guilford Press, New York, pp. 7-18.
Casper, C. R. (1983), On the emergence of bulimia nervosa as a syndrome: A historical view. *Int. J. Eating Disorders, 2*, 3-16.
Geist, R. A. (1984), Therapeutic dilemmas in the treatment of anorexia nervosa: A self psychological perspective. *Contemp. Psychother. Rev., 2*, 115-142.
Goldberg, A. (1983), On the scientific status of empathy. *Annual of Psychoanalysis, 11*, 155-170.
Goodsitt, A. (1983), Self regulatory disturbances in eating disorders. *Int. J. Eating Disorders, 3*, 51-60.
Goodsitt, A. (1985), Self psychology and the treatment of anorexia nervosa, in D. M. Garner and P. E. Garfinkel (Eds.), *Handbook of Psychotherapy for Anorexia Nervosa and Bulimia*, Guilford Press, New York, pp. 55-82.
Green, A. (1973), Introduction to the discussion on the genetic point of view. Unpublished manuscript.
Khan, M. (1978), Secret as potential space, in S. Grolnick and L. Barkin, *Reality and Fantasy*, Jason Aronson, New York, pp. 259-270.
Kohut, H. (1980), Reflections on advances in self psychology, in A. Goldberg, *Advances in Self Psychology*, International Universities Press, New York, pp. 473-554.
Kohut, H. (1984), *How Does Analysis Cure*, University of Chicago Press, Chicago.
Lerner, H. D. (1983), Contemporary psychoanalytic perspectives on gorge vomiting: A case illustration, *Int. J. Eating Disorders, 3*, 47-63.
Sugarman, A., and Kurash, C. (1982), The body as a transitional object in bulimia, *Int. J. Eating Disorders, 1*, 57-67.
Swift, W. J., and Letven, R. (1984), Bulimia and the basic fault: A psychoanalytic interpretation of the binging vomiting syndrome, *J. Am. Acad. Child Psychiatry, 23*, 483-497.
Tolpin, M. (1978), Selfobjects and oedipal objects: A crucial developmental distinction, *Psychoanal. Study Child, 33*, 167-184.
Tolpin, M. (1980), Discussion of "Psychoanalytic developmental theories of the self: An integration" by Morton Shane and Estelle Shane, in A. Goldberg (Ed.), *Advances in Self Psychology*, International Universities Press, New York, pp. 47-68.
Tolpin, M. (1983), Corrective emotional experience: A self psychological

re-evaluation, in A. Goldberg (Ed.), *The Future of Psychoanalysis*, International Universities Press, New York, pp. 363–380.
Winnicott, D. W. (1974), Fear of breakdown, *Int. Rev. Psychoanal., 1*, 97–106.
Wolf, E. (1980), On the developmental line of selfobject relations, in A. Goldberg (Ed.), *Advances in Self Psychology*, International Universities Press, New York, pp. 117–132.
Wolf, E. (1983), Empathy and countertransference, in A. Goldberg (Ed.), *The Future of Psychoanalysis*, International Universities Press, New York, pp. 309–326.

Massachusettes General Hospital
Department of Psychiatry, WACC-6
Boston, MA 02114

THE PARENTS' RELATIONSHIP AND THE CHILD'S ILLNESS IN ANOREXIA NERVOSA

CHRISTOPHER GORDON, M.D.
EUGENE BERESIN, M.D.
DAVID B. HERZOG, M.D.

The authors examine the impact on the preanorexic child of the parents' relationship with one another, particularly the models they present of mature male/female relationships. The authors suggest that patterns of maternal perfectionism and self-sacrifice combined with paternal entitlement makes sexual maturity particularly threatening for female children in these families, and may partially explain the greater incidence of anorexia nervosa in women, and its explosive incidence in adolescence.

One of the most striking aspects of anorexia nervosa is its tendency to afflict women. The disease affects women ten times more frequently than men, and tends to erupt at times of sexual maturation: menarche, puberty, and the development of a mature female body shape. There seems to be something about femininity that is particularly susceptible to anorexia, but unfortunately that something remains arcane. Most authors have ascribed this skewed distribution of the disease to the greater cultural press toward thinness in women and to differences in male and female experiences in puberty and adolescence (Garner et al., 1983). In this paper we will focus instead on what may be an additional important factor: the manner in which the parents of the anorexic child model male and female behavior, particularly on how the role of women is manifested in their relationship, and the corrosive consequences for the female child.

From the Department of Psychiatry, Massachusetts General Hospital. The authors gratefully acknowledge the critical assistance of Drs. Jules Bemporad, Catherine Steiner-Adair, and Paul Hamburg, and Julie Gordon, LICSW, in the preparation of this manuscript.

Crisp (1983), Minuchin et al. (1978), Palazzoli (1978), and Bemporad and Ratey (1985) have all noted that in many families with an anorexic child, the parental relationship is deeply troubled by mutual difficulties in intimacy and trust, but masked by a facade of smooth functioning, family loyalty, and solidarity. These and other authors have suggested that the anorexic child's illness acts to stabilize and protect the parental relationship. In confirming these observations, we have noted that parental conflicts often involve patterns of interaction that present frightening models of male/female behavior to the children, and seem to be especially noxious to the growth and development of female children.

As Bruch (1973), Palazzoli (1978), and Bemporad and Ratey (1985), among others, have noted, in one pattern common in many anorexics' families, the daughter's self-denial, rigidity, and perfectionism reflect similar values in her mother. In these families, mother is typically extraordinarily giving, attentive to the needs of everyone in the family, and perfectionistic in her strict standards for her own behavior, yet she is inhibited in directly asserting her own needs. She is more comfortable meeting the needs of others, and regards self-sacrifice as the highest virtue. She communicates an ideal of womanhood as selfless and unindulgent of appetites of any sort. Underneath her deference and solicitude to others, particularly to her husband, one senses impatience and resentment that are not expressed, since to express such feelings would be self-indulgent. Often she is married to a man who is as unable to give of himself as his wife is unable to take for herself. The husband, uneasy with dependency on women, assuages his distrust of women by devaluing them and by demanding unquestioning loyalty and deference from his wife and children. Frequently, however, the father's demands are covered over by an attitude of self-sacrifice or overwork. Both parents' needs are then obscured by apparent service to others.

In this sort of family structure, both parents' conflicts around dependency and intimacy become played out in their marital relationship. Both husband and wife are insulated against overwhelming closeness and dependency by virtue of this arrangement, yet both present models of adulthood that make female sexual maturity seem frightening and undesirable, since being a woman seems to imply being subordinate and unempowered in a world of powerful and demanding men. The daughter's intense loyalty to her mother, however, as well as the family's emphasis on outward harmony and solidarity, blocks her openly questioning her mother's behavior; her identification with mother blocks her questioning her father's behavior. The child — particularly the female child — is caught in a double-bind.

We have observed this pattern of maternal perfectionism and paternal entitlement with great regularity in our anorexic patients. There are many variations, for example, the mother may put much more overt pressure on the child in an almost "show business mother" fashion, or the father may be more or less overtly entitled. The family features we wish to underscore are the subordination of the child's needs to the parents' needs for performance from the child, and the enactment in the parental relationship of mutual inauthenticity and distrust that make the world seem a dangerous place, particularly for women.

We do not believe that these dynamics underlie all cases of anorexia nervosa, and we understand that it is erroneous to over-generalize about anorexics and their families. We appreciate that much of the apparent psychopathology one observes in these families may well be more a result than a cause of the disease (Yager, 1982). Our observations are based on interviews with anorexics, their parents, and families. We have treated approximately 50 anorexic patients in the last 10 years, and have supervised the treatment of perhaps twice that number. Since we feel that this pattern has significance for the treatment of many of these women, we believe it is well worth bearing in mind, even if it does not apply to every anorexic or to every family.

The pattern of family dynamics we examine in this paper offers a new perspective on several pieces of the anorexia nervosa puzzle: the lack of empathy felt by the daughter of a mother who is, overtly, conscientious; the role of sexuality, pseudosexuality, and competition with mother in dealing with father and other males; the crisis presented by puberty and adolescence; the relative invulnerability of sons to anorexia; and the implacable resistance of the anorexic patient to the interventions of family or therapist.

THE DYNAMIC BASIS OF
ANOREXIA NERVOSA

Previous authors have not emphasized the role of the parental representation of male/female relationships in the development of anorexia nervosa. Instead, attention has primarily been focused on the relationship with mother and the sense of self in anorexia nervosa. Hilde Bruch (1982) hypothesized that gratifying early experiences with feeding instill in the infant a sense of confidence, both about the accuracy of her interoceptive sensations of hunger and other appetites and in the availability of the mother to respond appropriately to her cues. Bruch argued that this connection with mother lays the foundation both for a sense of coherent self and a sense of trust in the world.

Bruch proposed that when appropriate responses from the mother are chronically lacking, such as when the mother feeds the child primarily out of her own needs to quiet the child or make her sleep, the child develops uncertainty about her ability to discriminate her inner states and a uneasiness about being able to contact her mother and elicit care. The anorexic-to-be trusts neither herself nor the world. She feels instead a desperate need to comply with what she construes to be her mother's needs, in order to maintain what feels like a frail connection with her mother. Hence the perfectionism, compliance, and desperation of the anorexic stance (Jeammet, 1981).

Palazzoli (1978) underscored a further, more complicated consequence of the failure in the relationship with mother: the child's inability to test out her hostility and aggression against a reliable and forgiving maternal presence. When the child feels she must absolutely comply with mother's wishes, her aggression and hostility must be renounced. In their renunciation they are projected onto the significant people around the child, largely onto mother, and the world is then even further colored by untrustworthiness: the child experiences the world as menacing rather than simply unempathic. The child's perception of her mother and the world as fundamentally hostile to her is both an expression of her dread and a way of maintaining object ties through hostile dependency. Hence the paranoid anticipation of "pouncing criticism" in anorexia nervosa (Bruch, 1973).

Another consequence of the disturbed relation with the mother is the attempt to preserve an image of the mother as a good object by idealization and splitting. Unable to integrate her own aggression and hostility, the child cannot integrate her mother's inevitable hostility either. Instead, the mother must be seen as perfect, ideal, and unsullied by anger, hostility, frustration, and other failings. While this idealization preserves for the child the possibility of a good object being in the world, it does so at great cost: the girl has a sense that the perfect, idealized mother is unpleasable; no one can measure up to her standards; her rage, submerged under an angelic demeanor, can only be guessed at but if awakened must be terrible; and horrid comparison of the faulty self with the maternal ideal is unbearable. Moreover, these unintegrated good and bad objects, once reintrojected, form the basis for pathologic, fantastic object relations that further impair the child's use of available objects in the real world. These reintrojected all-good; all-bad objects provide prototypes for the savage, primitive superego precursors that plague anorexic individuals in the place of mature superego structures and the ego ideal (Kernberg, 1975).

Hence the anorexic child from an object relations perspective is fixated at a developmental level that antedates the consolidation of trust. She is incapable of either genuine concern for another person or belief in another's concern for her. Her sense of self is fragile and unreliable. Having been unable to integrate her own aggression, she experiences it projected all around her as a hostile world and within in her as terrible primitive rage and equally unmodulated guilt. In the anorexic's world, something terrible is always about to happen. Any good thing—her mother's love, her mother's approval, any achievement the child may possess—seems always on the verge of turning into its opposite. She fends off these disasters and finds her way in the world by relying on formulas, concrete and magical algorithms of what is right and good, to deal with people she perceives as fundamentally untrustworthy and unforgiving.

These formulations, based on Bruch's seminal observations, illuminate the self-sustaining interaction between empathic failure, pathologic object relations, and schizoid avoidance of human relationships in anorexia nervosa. Each factor reinforces and increases the need for the others. Together they largely preclude new, satisfying, and growth-promoting experiences in the world, yielding a closed circle of stagnant redundancy, constriction of experience, and emotional shallowness. This synergistic interaction between the child's intrapsychic structure and her experience of receiving inadequate empathy from the family environment also helps to explain the anorexic's formidable resistance to parental pressure to change, as well as her often insurmountable resistance to psychotherapy. The anorexia nervosa is at once a desperate attempt to be what mother seems to want and at the same time a hostile-dependent expression of rage and protest.

PRECOCIOUS OEDIPALITY AND
ANOREXIA NERVOSA

The anorexic child's tendency to view the world as dangerous is compounded by her attitude toward sexuality. The anorexic adolescent presents an amalgam of intense dread of sexuality in herself and others intermixed with a tendency to oversexualize relationships, people, and objects. She may be seductive and flirtatious, provocative and exhibitionistic, or may appear intensely phobic about all things sexual. In either case, the anorexic woman exists not merely in a frightening world, but a world imbued with terrifying sexuality.

Kernberg (1980) from an object relations perspective, and Geist (1984) from a self-psychological one, have shed important light on this aspect of anorexia. Kernberg, discussing borderline personality structures, demonstrates how failures in early dyadic relations with the mother lead the child to turn toward the father to meet emotional needs. This precocious push into oedipal relations is fueled by two needs: first to escape the all-bad part-object mother (as the child sees her); and second, to find mothering in the oedipal relationship with the father. This pseudo-sexual oedipal advance, however, pits the child against her mother and increases her anxiety.

Geist (1984) has specifically addressed these issues in anorexia nervosa. Arguing that maternal failures in empathy lead to a pathological tendency in the child toward slavish compliance with the mother's needs for a perfect child, Geist sees the anorexic child's turning toward her father primarily as a search for the mirroring admiration and empathy that were lacking in the maternal relation. Geist believes that sexual maturation in adolescence threatens this father-daughter closeness, and may partially explain the eruption of anorexia nervosa in the parapubertal period.

Whether from an object relations or self-psychological perspective, this tendency toward precocious, pseudosexual oedipal strivings places the child in a precarious position of competition with her mother, the same mother to whom she is slavishly devoted, to whom her compliance is dedicated, and whose rage and wrath the child almost never experiences (being such a "good girl"), but imagines as terrible in scope and irreparable in consequences.

FAMILY STRUCTURE IN ANOREXIA NERVOSA

The family structure of many anorexics compounds the child's sense of uneasiness. Minuchin et al. (1975) have observed that the child in many such families does in fact occupy a triangulated position between her parents. These families often appear to be deeply in conflict, with separation of the parents a recurrent veiled or real threat (Kalucy et al., 1977). These conflicts are rarely directly acknowledged or resolved but are frequently "detoured" through the symptomatic child (Minuchin et al, 1975). As Crisp (1983) has pointed out, often the maturation of this symptomatic child threatens the balance of the family system. Such a position in the family reinforces the anorexic girl's sense of insecurity, distrust, hyperresponsiblity, and fears regarding male-female mating and sexuality.

But how do such family dynamics develop? These are hardly neglectful families. As Palazzoli (1978) has observed most of these mothers are exquisitely concerned, both about their daughters and their whole families. To the extent that feminine identity centers on valuing the self and others through interdependent relationships, as Gilligan (1982) has recently argued, the mother may seem to embody feminine relatedness.

However, on closer inspection, in most of these mothers' relationships, underneath the apparent attention to the family's needs, one usually senses a distinctively defensive need to be "good" and to meet the needs of others to the exclusion of her own. Indeed in our and others' observations, the mothers of many anorexic patients have an almost martyred role in the family and often despite external achievements seem markedly deficient in self-esteem. Like her anorexic child's compliance, it is as though mother's generosity, deferentiality, and solicitude were meant to make up for an internal sense of badness or inadequacy. As it is for the anorexic child, the appearance of goodness, of being above reproach in the eyes of others, is of paramount importance. Like her anorexic daughter's frenzied feeding of others while she herself starves, much of the mother's apparent generosity proceeds not so much from a sense of genuine concern about the needs of the other person, but rather in order to control or undo unacceptable aspects of the self. The mother's behavior signifies a frightening distortion of mature femininity: what looks like relatedness conceals distrust; apparent generosity conceals a sense of selfishness and worthlessness; and apparent concern covers a need to control.

Maternal Reactive Generosity

Kernberg (1980) has termed this kind of giving to others "reactive generosity," proceeding in reaction to an internal sense of badness, guilt, and projected hostility. Reactive generosity differs from authentic generosity, which springs from normal reparative guilt and empathic concern. The mother's reactive generosity usually has two important targets. First, the mothers we are describing here are usually quite deferential and solicitous to their husbands, sometimes to the point of servility. Not surprisingly, one often senses beneath the surface anger and contempt at having to defer, but these unacceptable affects are managed by further reactive attentiveness and "good works." In fact, the undoing of these unwanted affects may be a major driving force maintaining the reactive generosity. The second major object of the mother's generosity is often her own mother. We have repeatedly observed that in families in which the mother displays this reactive generosity, she usually feels that her own selflessness pales beside her own mother's goodness and near saintliness. No matter how giving or selfless the mother may appear, she usually reports feeling not good enough, particularly in comparison with her own mother, to whom her attempts at perfection (including trying to have perfect children) are a sort of tribute. This sense of inferiority to her mother is of course at the center of the anorexic girl's experience as well, a paradoxical common bond with her own mother. Not surprisingly, in many of these mothers we observe subclinical anorexia, a *forme fruste* in the second generation.

The mother's reactive generosity makes for other problems for the child. Being the recipient of the mother's reactive generosity is a disquieting and confusing experience. Reactive generosity is not attuned to the needs of the recipient, but to the needs of the giver. The giver of reactive generosity needs the recipient to be in need, and cannot tolerate the recipient giving in her turn. Receiving gifts that are born out of reactive generosity engenders not gratification and gratitude but perplexity. There is no right way to receive such gifts. If one accepts gratefully, one feels somehow wrong; after all, mother does not take such gifts. If on the other hand, one refuses, one feels wrong; after all, mother is only trying to be kind. In place of gratification and gratitude, the recipient feels guilt, confusion, and a need both to comply and not to comply with the mother's wishes. This is of course precisely what occurs in anorexia: the girl becomes the quintessential good girl, so good that she is infuriating in her self-denial and yet seems above reproach.

An additional aspect of the mother's perfectionism and emphasis on being "good" is that while she is often demanding and controlling toward her children and others, usually her demands are presented not as her own needs or wishes but as "right," "proper," or admirable behaviors. The mother controls by the induction of guilt, often disguising her needs (for example, for the appearance of a perfect family) as concern for the other person. The mother's hidden agenda powerfully confirms the anorexic child's sense that things are not as they seem, that despite apparent acceptance and support from others, terrible criticism may erupt at any time.

All in all, the mother's behavior and world view share many features with her anorexic daughter's. The anorexic child's self-starvation and perfectionism are distortions of normal self-control; however, they simulate normal self-control sufficiently closely that they are not ego-alien to the patient, nor, often for a long time, to family and friends (Branch and Eurman, 1980). The mother's reactive generosity is a distortion of normal empathy and feminine relatedness, nearly into their opposites, yet her behavior so closely simulates empathic relatedness that it is perplexing to others and even to the mother herself. Her reactive generosity laced with distrust of men represents a disturbing model of femininity. Her behavior seems to imply that being a woman with a man means subjugating herself to him rather than being interdependent with him; the mother's disguised contempt and distrust of men convey that there is much to be feared and avoided in the world of sexual maturity.

Paternal Narcissistic Entitlement

In many families we have seen, the mother's deferentiality, solicitude, and apparent generosity are matched by a complementary entitlement to this behavior in the father. In some fathers this takes the form of autocracy in decision making, ruling the family unilaterally; in others it may take even more blatant forms, such as demanding the largest or best serving of food. Many of these fathers are extremely successful in their professional lives where indeed they may rule with just this sort of authority. One frequently discerns beneath the professional success and mastery of these men problems in self-esteem and basic trust that are similar to their wives' issues: a needy, dependent, and frightened side, which is fiercely denied. These men distrust women, who are perceived as powerful in their capacity to betray and abandon, and often deal with their distrust by attempts to control and dominate women.

These husbands are exquisitely sensitive to hidden resentment and hostility beneath their wives' reactive generosity. Again like their wives, these fathers often do not consciously acknowledge their needs, nor are they often confronted by their wives—at least those whom we are describing here—because their own deferentiality proscribes such self-assertion.

The father's attitude toward women contributes to the difficulties of the female child's oedipal strivings. In the father's ongoing struggle with his wife, he may see his adoring, oedipal daughter as delightfully, reassuringly safe: the child cannot abandon him, and her childish idealization and adoration may closely approximate what he is seeking in relations with women generally. Consequently he may reciprocate his daughter's oedipal interest in a frightening way; oedipal victory may seem all too possible. Excessive closeness with the father compounds the sense of uneasiness communicated by the mother, and seems to confirm the mother's view of the male world as dangerous. Moreover, the child feels drawn into competition with the very person with whose wishes she is trying desperately to comply.

Just as the mother's behavior is a distortion of feminine relatedness, the father's behavior is a distortion and exaggeration of masculine strength into narcissistic isolation, autocracy, and misogyny. The father's entitlement confirms and underscores the child's impression that dependence on a man means subjugation to him, that there is much to be avoided and dreaded in the world of men.

Thus, the parents are narcissistically isolated from each other, each having problems of intimacy and trust, yet remaining involved and engaged with one another in a self-sustaining cycle: the father has a sense that beneath his wife's solicitude there lurks a terrible anger and contempt, which is just what he expects from powerful women; the mother repeatedly experiences her husband as infantile, explosive, and capricious—in need of just the sort of deference she offers, and just as deserving of her hidden contempt. This cycle, usually concealed under a facade of smooth functioning, preserves both parents from the twin dangers of excessive closeness on the one hand and abandonment on the other. The parents are paradoxically comforted and stabilized by their mutual distrust. But the ways in which they enact their distrust—particularly the ways in which they present role models of men and women—have profound consequences for their children, especially their daughters.

IMPLICATIONS FOR THE CHILD

Understanding the child's perceptions of her parents' relationship, and her place in it, sheds light on two important aspects of anorexia nervosa: its tendency to erupt in adolescence and its markedly greater incidence in girls than in boys. For the anorexic-to-be, the onset of puberty and menarche are profoundly disturbing. Her shaky sense of self-esteem and her intense need to comply with her mother's wishes make separation from the family threatening. Her fearful anticipation of criticism, rigid formulas, and black-and-white thinking compromise her ability to join the tumultuous peer group of other adolescents. The world seems unmanageable, hostile — she has no place to be safe.

But even more disturbing than separation from her mother in adolescence are the pulls toward her, in an increasing sense of identification with her as the body matures. As the girl's body seems to be becoming more and more like her mother's, the lack of adequate role models in both father and mother of adults who can be simultaneously interdependent and autonomous becomes crucial. The transformation of the body, and the pull of the sexual appetites feel to the child like she will of necessity become a woman in her mother's mold, and pulled toward a man in her father's image. Dependency will equal slavery; intimacy will mean surrendering integrity; sexuality will mean a loss of control over her own appetites and a man's appetites; and all of this will mean renunciation of her only sense of safety at all: her sense of being her mother's child.

The girl's relationship with her mother and father give her little comfort as she takes on the role of young adult in her family. The relationship with her mother has been based on the child's compliance with her mother's need for a perfect child; in the face of multiplying appetites and urges and the normal adolescent impulse toward rebelliousness and dysphoria, the relationship with her mother offers no guidelines. Her father's attitude toward adult women makes female maturity a frightening prospect. For the anorexic-to-be the solution is the reversal of adolescence, separation, and mature sexuality by self-starvation.

Why is the female child more sensitive to the problems in the family than are sons? One possibility is that the values that the mother appears to be espousing — service to others, concern for the other, attention to the relationship — are very close to the girl's innate inclinations toward making and sustaining relationships and for having empathy for those with whom the relationships are made. As Gilligan (1982) has demonstrated this interrelatedness lies at the center of feminine development, more so than it does for boys, who tend to be more autonomous, self-directed, and rule-oriented in their relationships with others, and who hew their sense of self out of renouncing ties to mother rather than sustaining a relationship with her. What the anorexic's mother seems to be modelling feels right and familiar to her female child. What is perplexing and in the end crippling is that the mother's emphasis on the needs of others is defensive and designed to cover feelings of inner inadequacy. She espouses concern but demonstrates an incapacity for empathy-in-depth, since from her daughter she seems to want imitation and compliance, not authentic response. The mother's behavior, then, is a sort of caricature of feminine concern. The daughter's inclination toward interrelatedness feels untrustworthy to her: interrelationship with her mother means subordination to her mother's wishes; interrelationship with men means subjugation to male egocentricity. Again there is no place to be safe.

For male children in these families, then, failures in the relationship with the mother are less threatening. The son is less empathically attuned to lapses in maternal empathy. When the mother-child dyad is threatened, the girl responds empathically to repair it — by compliance if necessary. In contrast, the boy who is faced with similar lapses in maternal empathy may respond with greater renunciation of ties to his mother and greater "autonomy" from her. This pattern of intensified renunciation of maternal ties would be expected to lead a male child into pathological narcissistic self-sufficiency and a distrustful misogynistic view of women generally — often precisely the model of manhood offered by his father.

From this perspective, anorexia nervosa can be seen in part as an expression of horror and protest against the girl's perception of her mother's life and fate; but it is a muffled, hidden, and encoded protest, as the girl tries to confirm, love, and idealize her mother at the same time. Anorexia nervosa may be seen as an attempt by the child to awaken her mother, to contact her, and to break her out of her own vicious cycle of self-sacrifice and self-denial, but without any appearance of rejecting the mother herself. The anorexia can be viewed as a caricature of the mother's version of womanhood. It is a desperate attempt to comply with the mother's standards and at the same time to question their very foundation.

In conclusion, we wish to reiterate that we do not believe that these dynamics underlie all cases of anorexia nervosa. We believe, however, that understanding the role of the parental relationship, and particularly the representation of the role and worth of women within it, sheds light on the predominance of anorexia nervosa in women and its tendency to erupt in adolescence.

References

Branch, C. H. H., and Eurman, L. J. (1980), Social attitudes toward patients with anorexia nervosa, *Am. J. Psychiatry, 137*, 631–632.

Bemporad, J. R., and Ratey, J. (1985), Intensive psychotherapy of former anorexic individuals, *Am. J. of Psychother., 39*, 454–465.

Bruch, H. (1973), *Eating Disorders: Obesity, Anorexia Nervosa, and the Person Within*, Basic Books, New York.

Bruch, H. (1982), Anorexia nervosa: Therapy and theory, *Am. J. Psychiatry, 139*, 1531–1538.

Crisp, A. H. (1983), *Anorexia Nervosa: Let Me Be*, Grune and Stratton, New York.

Garner, D. M., Garfinkel, P. E., and Olmstead, M. P. (1983), An overview of sociocultural factors in the development of anorexia nervosa, in *Anorexia Nervosa: Recent Developments in Research*, Alan R. Liss, New York, pp. 65–82.

Geist, R. A. (1984), Psychotherapeutic dilemmas in the treatment of anorexia nervosa: A self-psychological perspective, *Contemp. Psychother. Rev., 2*, 268–288.

Gilligan, C. (1982), *In a Different Voice*, Harvard University Press, Cambridge.

Jeammet, P. (1981), The anorexic stance, *J. Adolescence, 4*, 113–129.

Kalucy, R. S., Crisp, A. H., and Harding, B. (1977), A study of 56 families with anorexia nervosa, *Br. J. Med. Psychol., 50*, 381–395.

Kernberg, O. (1975), *Borderline Conditions and Pathological Narcissism*, Jason Aronson, New York.

Kernberg, O. (1980), Melanie Klein, in H. I. Kaplan, A. M. Freedman, and B. J. Sadoch (Eds.), *Comprehensive Textbook of Psychiatry III*, Williams and Wilkins, Baltimore, pp. 820–833.

Minuchin, S., Baker, L., Rosman, B. L., Liebman, R., Milman, L., and Todd, T. (1975), A conceptual model of psychodynamic illness in children, *Arch. Gen. Psychiatry, 32*, 1031–1038.

Minuchin, S., Rosman, B. L., and Baker, L. (1978), *Psychosomatic Families*, Harvard University Press, Cambridge.
Palazzoli, M. S. (1982), *Self-Starvation*, Jason Aronson, New York.
Yager, J. (1982), Family issues in the pathogenesis of anorexia nervosa, *Psychosom. Med., 44*, 43–60.

227 Babcock Street
Brookline, MA 02146

INFANTILE ANOREXIA NERVOSA: A DEVELOPMENTAL DISORDER OF SEPARATION AND INDIVIDUATION

IRENE CHATOOR, M.D.

Infantile anorexia nervosa is an eating disorder that has its onset during the early developmental stage of separation and individuation between the ages of six months and three years. Infantile anorexia nervosa is characterized by food refusal and leads to failure to thrive. The infant refuses to eat in an attempt to achieve autonomy and control with regard to the mother, a maneuver that serves to involve the mother more deeply in the infant's eating behavior and to meet the infant's need for attention. Mother and infant become embroiled in a battle of wills over the infant's food intake. The infant's feeding is directed by his emotional needs instead of physiological sensations of hunger and satiety, and he fails to develop somatopsychological differentiation. The infant's temperament and maternal conflicts over control, autonomy, and dependency appear to contribute to this eating disorder. Treatment is aimed toward helping the parents understand and promote the developmental process of somatopsychological differentiation. Initially, a behavioral–cognitive approach is used; however, parents who struggle with unresolved issues around dependency and control require further psychotherapy.

INTRODUCTION

Infantile anorexia nervosa, an eating disorder of infants and young children, was first described as a separation disorder by Egan et al. (1980) and by Chatoor and Egan (1983). Although it usually leads to growth failure, infantile anorexia nervosa was not

Irene Chatoor is Associate Professor, Psychiatry and Behavioral Sciences, and Child Health and Development, George Washington University, School of Medicine; Psychiatric Director of Psychosomatic and Eating Disorders Program, Children's Hospital National Medical Center.

previously recognized as a specific type of failure to thrive. The diagnosis of failure to thrive is most commonly made when the child's decelerated or arrested growth results in weight and height measurements that fall below the third percentiles on the Boston Growth Standards or demonstrate a persistent deviation below the established growth curve, across two major percentiles over time (Woolston, 1985).

Failure to thrive is a serious, complex disorder of multiple etiologies that afflicts infants and children. One feature frequently found in all varieties of failure to thrive is the occurrence of feeding problems. The variety of feeding problems and the specificity of certain feeding difficulties at different ages has led to our developmental classification of feeding disorders (Chatoor et al. 1984, 1985; Chatoor and Egan, 1987). Anna Freud (1946) first drew attention to the developmental aspects of feeding problems and postulated a developmental line from suckling to rational eating. Our classification of feeding disturbances incorporates Greenspan and Lourie's (1981) stages of early infant development and Mahler et al.'s (1975) concepts of separation and individuation. We differentiate three distinct stages of feeding development during which adaptive and maladaptive behaviors can be observed in both the mother and the infant. Disorders of homeostasis occur in the first two months of life, disorders of attachment between the ages of two and six months, and disorders of separation or infantile anorexia nervosa between six months and three years of age. In our view each of these three developmental feeding disorders can create, exacerbate, or be a sequela of failure to thrive.

DIAGNOSIS

Infantile anorexia nervosa usually begins between six months and three years of age, during the developmental phase of separation and individuation (Mahler et al., 1975). Both motoric and cognitive development enable the infant to function with more emotional independence. As the infant begins to crawl away from the mother, he becomes increasingly aware of his separateness and must confront the developmental issues of autonomy versus dependency. His new cognitive capacities allow him to understand the relationship between cause and effect and he becomes aware that his actions elicit certain reactions from his caretakers. This awareness becomes evident in the increasing intentionality and willfulness observed during this period of development. Part of this learning process involves somatopsychological differentiation (Greenspan and Lieberman, 1981). The infant begins to understand and differentiate a variety of somatic sensations, such as hunger, satiety or tiredness, from emotional feelings such as anger, frustration or need for affection. As with the earlier developmental stages, both partners of the dyad contribute to the successful resolution of this process: the infant, by clearly signaling his somatic versus his emotional needs; the caretaker, by reading the infant's signals correctly and by responding in a contingent manner. For example, when the infant cries the mother then must determine whether the infant is hungry or tired or in need of comfort and affection. Her response has to address the infant's expression of his specific need. When the infant stops eating the mother must determine whether the infant is feeling sated, seeking attention, or expressing anger and refusing her food in protest.

Infantile anorexia nervosa is characterized by failure to thrive and food refusal or extreme food selectivity and undereating despite efforts by the parents to increase the infant's food intake. Characteristically the parents mention that they have tried "everything" to induce the infant to eat, which usually means coaxing, cajoling, bargaining, distracting, or forcing food into the infant's mouth. These parental responses interfere with the development of somatopsychological differentiation.

BACKGROUND STUDIES

To better understand the interactional patterns of mothers and infants with infantile anorexia nervosa and how they differ from those of mothers and infants without any feeding problems, Chatoor et al. (1988) studied 42 infants and toddlers with infantile anorexia nervosa and 30 control subjects matched for age, sex, and race. The average age of the infants at onset of the study was 20 months. According to Hollingshead's criteria, 30 infants were from an upper socioeconomic environment and 12 infants were from a lower one; 28 were caucasian and 14 were black; 22 were female and 20 were male.

All 72 infants and toddlers were videotaped from behind a one-way mirror in two adjacent hospital offices during a 20-minute feeding period followed by a 10-minute play period. Trained observers rated the videotapes with global rating scales for feeding and for play developed by Chatoor et al. (1984b, 1985b). These scales utilize a four-point Likert-type format for rating the behavior and affect of mother–infant pairs.

T-tests for each subscale from the Feeding Scale revealed significant differences between the groups of infants with infantile anorexia nervosa and the control group on four out of five subscales. Whereas the control group showed better dyadic reciprocity, the interactions of the feeding disordered group were characterized by more conflict, more struggle for control, and more maternal noncontingency. Although there was a subgroup within the infants with infantile anorexia nervosa who scored highly on "bargaining about food" and who showed better reciprocity than the rest, overall group variation on this subscale was not statistically significant.

T-tests between the feeding disordered and the control group for each item on the Feeding Scale demonstrated significant group differences for 35 of the 46 mother and infant behaviors (Table 1).

The Play Scale revealed similar results. *T*-tests between the eating-disordered and control group revealed significant differences between the groups on all four subscales. The feeding-disordered group showed less dyadic reciprocity and more conflict. The mothers scored higher on unresponsiveness to the infant's needs on one hand and on intrusiveness on the other hand. *T*-tests between the eating-disordered and the control groups for each item revealed that 20 out of 32 items were significantly different for the two groups (Table 2).

These results are striking in that the mothers and infants of the feeding-disordered group clearly lacked the reciprocal exchange observed in the control group. The mothers of the infants with infantile anorexia nervosa appeared more self-directed and controlling as evidenced by their missing and overriding the infant's signals. These mothers and infants appeared to be out of step with one another during their interactions. However, the mother's negative affect of anger, frustration, and sadness was mirrored by her infant's affect.

Bruch (1973) and Palazzoli (1974) have postulated that dysfunctioning in the mother–infant relationship underlies the development of anorexia nervosa during adolescence. From detailed reconstruction of the developmental histories of her patients, Bruch concluded that "there was a paucity of appropriate and confirming responses by the parent to signals indicating the child's needs and other forms of self expression" (p. 55). Bruch postulated that appropriate responses to cues coming from the infant, in the biologi-

Table 1.   Items from the Feeding Scale Showing Significant ($p < .05$) Differences between Feeding Disordered and Control Group

---

Mother (Control group scored better than feeding-disordered group)

Positions infant for reciprocal exchange
Talks to infant
Waits for infant to initiate interactions
Shows pleasure toward infant in gaze, voice, or smile
Makes positive remarks to infant
Makes positive statements about infant's food intake or food preferences
Appears cheerful
Positions infant without regard for needed support
Positions or holds infant with restriction of normal movement
Handles infant in abrupt or rough manner
Acts erratically of inconsistently
Makes negative or critical statements to infant
Tells infant to eat, to do, or not to do
Makes negative or critical statements about infant's food intake or food
   preferences
Misses infant's cues
Controls feeding by overriding infant's cues
Forces bottle or food into infant's mouth
Appears sad
Appears distressed
Appears angry

Infant (control group scored better than feeding-disordered group)

Looks at mother
Smiles at mother
Vocalizes to mother
Appears cheerful
Avoids gaze
Stiffens when touched or held
Appears easily distracted away from feeding
Cries when food offered
Pushes food away or throws food
Refuses to open mouth
Turns away from food
Arches from food
Spits food out
Appears angry
Appears distressed

Table 2.   Items from Play Scale Showing Significant ($p<.05$) Differences between Feeding-Disordered and Control Group

---

Mother (Control group scored better than feeding-disordered group)

Positions infant for reciprocal exchange
Waits for infant to initiate interactions
Shows pleasure toward infant in gaze, voice, or smile
Makes encouraging positive remarks about infant's play
Engages in pleasurable give and take with infant during play
Attends to infant's play with interest and pleasure
Appears cheerful
Handles infant in abrupt or rough manner
Makes negative or critical statements to infant
Directs infant to do or not to do
Controls infant's play without regard for infant's cues
Appears oblivious to infant's activity
Appears sad
Appears detached
Appears distressed

Infant (control group scored better than feeding-disordered group)

Looks at mother
Plays with mother
Appears cheerful
Avoids gaze
Appears angry

---

cal as well as in the intellectual, social, and emotional field are necessary for the child to organize the significant building blocks for development of self-awareness and self-effectiveness. If a mother's reactions are continuously inappropriate, neglectful, oversolicitous, inhibiting, or indiscriminately permissive, the child will experience confusion. Rizzuto et al. (1981) also propose that the abnormal development of the anorectic adolescent is caused by the mother's inability to reflect back to the baby the baby's own self, her inability to fulfill the mirror role of the mother as proposed by Winnicott (1971).

This lack of mirroring and inability to read and to respond to the infant's cues was the most salient feature of the mothers of the eating-disordered infants in the study on mother–infant interactions by Chatoor et al. (1988) previously described. In interviews, we discovered that these mothers had good intentions and high expectations of themselves in their role as mother. They were very distressed by their infants' oppositional behaviors and food refusal and unsure of how to change these behaviors. These mothers were uncomfortable with and tended to repress negative feelings toward the infant. A few mothers admitted to feelings of such intense anger and frustration that they sometimes had feared losing control and hurting the infant. It appeared that their guilty feelings about wanting to abandon or hurt the infant lead to the mothers' increased efforts to be "a good mother" and to their inability to set appropriate limits to their infants' increasing demands and provocative behaviors. Eventually, these mothers could no longer contain their angry feelings. Their repressed anger would either seem to paralyze them or lead to forcefeeding or other examples of forceful punishment of the infants. These incidents of overt anger were experienced by the mothers as loss of control, "being a bad mother." The mothers would set a new cycle into motion by making up to the infant and being extra lenient and loving. Thus, these mothers were inconsistent and extreme in their responses to the infant. Their responses seemed largely governed not by the behaviors initiated by the infant but by the mother's internal state.

During treatment two major groups of mothers emerged who seemed unable to successfully negotiate issues of autonomy versus dependency with their infants during this developmental phase of separation and individuation.

One group of mothers seemed to be more comfortable with the infant's autonomy during play but had developed a "blind spot" when dealing with the infant during feeding. These dyads had usually experienced some transient feeding difficulties when the infant was ill, which seemed to have "sensitized" the mother to worry excessively about the infant's growth. These mothers seemed to feel insecure in their mother role and measured their competence by how well the infant ate. Because of high anxiety during feeding, these mothers were unable to read the infant's cues correctly. Feeding became an increasingly frustrating task as the toddler refused to eat in an effort to assert more autonomy and control.

Another group of mothers reported intense conflicts with their own mothers during their growing years, which had continued into the adult years. They had been informed of poor childhood eating behaviors by their mothers or remembered their own battles, over food during childhood and over money in their adults years. One mother illustrated her mother's attitude very eloquently: "My mother was so restrictive and controlling, she blocked out the sun during my childhood, and she gives me a pounding headache for two days whenever she calls now." These young mothers appeared to make conscious efforts to be loving and caring toward their infants. They had trouble tolerating their own negative or angry feelings toward their infants because those feelings represented "being like my mother." They wanted to be better mothers than the model of their own mothers, but "the ghosts from their nursery" to use Frailberg et al.'s (1975) apt phrase, continued to intrude in their relationship with their infants. Their own conflicts around autonomy and control in their relationship with their mothers were reactivated when their infants entered the developmental phase of separation and individuation.

Most mothers reported a blissful period in their relationship with their infants in the first six months of life when the infant was most dependent, passive, and compliant. However, with the emergence of new cognitive and motoric skills, when the infants began to express their own wills and demonstrated oppositional behaviors in an attempt to separate from mother, the mothers appeared unequipped to negotiate increasing autonomy with their infants and to set appropriate limits to unacceptable behaviors. They did not want to be the harsh, punitive mother that they had experienced in their own mothers, but they lacked the emotional experience of alternative role models. In order to be the caring and understanding mother they had yearned for during their childhood, these mothers exerted great effort to feed their infants. They appeared unable to recognize the infant's grabbing for the spoon or holding on to the dish as efforts at autonomy and self-feeding. They appeared overdetermined to feed the infant and to control the feeding believing they were most effective in getting food into the infant's mouth. When the infants refused to open their mouths, cried or arched their backs in protest, the mothers were unable to interpret these behaviors correctly; instead they felt frustrated and rejected by the infants. They then exerted even greater efforts, bargaining, begging, and distracting the infants. However, the more effort expanded the more resistant the infants became to eating mother's way and the more skillful they grew in eliciting mother's attention by refusing to eat.

Although most mother–infant dynamics fit these two categories, other interactions indicated variations in conflict over issues of autonomy versus dependency. Further research is required to better understand the spectrum of psychopathology in the mothers and how maternal conflicts impact on the infant's feeding behavior.

The fathers of the infants with this eating disorder presented a varied picture. In some cases they were intimately involved in the care of the infants, and were, also drawn into the infant's battles over food. In other cases, the fathers were physically or emotionally removed from the family and left the care of the infants almost completely to the mother. In a number of cases there was intense conflict between the parents with the infant's food refusal being at the center of parental disagreement. It appears that the father's psychopathology and involvement with the mother and the infant are important variables that also determine the severity of the separation difficulties and eating disorder of the infant. Experience in offspring studies of affective disorders reveal that the mother's affective psychopathology may be either neutralized or intensified by the father's mental functioning as well as his involvement in child-rearing processes. Further research should focus on the role of the father in mitigating or intensifying the infant's conflict around autonomy and control and the development of the eating disorder.

A key finding of infant research has been the discovery of the infant as an active partner in transactions with adults. However, the degree to which the infant controls the interactional process as contrasted to how much he passively surrenders to the adult seems to vary greatly depending upon the situation and the individual infant's temperament. One striking observation of infants with infantile anorexia nervosa is their willfulness. They are persistent, and frequently forceful or provocative in the expression of their wants. They seem to watch and study their mothers carefully. They appear to anticipate their mother's reactions and display an "I dare you mother" attitude. These temperamental characteristics are in strong contrast to those of the toddler who becomes anorectic during adolescence, usually remembered as the "best little child." The parents of these youngsters usually do not remember any oppositional behaviors during the early years of development. They recall only pleasing compliance when they think of the growing years of their adolescent anorectic. The adolescent anorectic appears to have had a talent for observing and anticipating the parents' responses and an ability to accommodate his/her own behavior accordingly. It appears that these temperamental differences result in early versus late onset of anorexia nervosa. The willful and demanding infant provokes a power struggle with the mother during the early phase of separation and individuation whereas the passivity and easy compliance of the adolescent anorectic allow a life as an extension of the mother until the demands of adolescence force a break from this symbiosis.

Both the infantile and the adolescent anorectic struggle with issues of separation and autonomy. In both situations, these conflicts affect eating behavior and interfere with the development of somatopsychological differentiation. This developmental process begins in the second half of the first year of life when the infant begins to understand basic schemes of causality. The mother facilitates this process by responding contingently to the infant's cues. As described previously in this paper the mother must differentiate between the infant's signals for food or for affection and must determine whether the infant is full or frustrated in his attempts at self-feeding. If the mother misses or repeatedly overrides the infant's cues, the infant becomes confused as to differences between physical sensations and emotional needs. For example, the mother misinterprets the infant's attempts at self-feeding and insists on feeding herself. Consequently, the infant may refuse to eat. The infant's food intake becomes controlled by anger and the need to assert himself rather than by feelings of hunger and fullness. On the other hand, if the mother disregards the infant's cues of satiety and attempts more feeding by distracting, playing games, or force-feeding, the infant learns that mother's affection or anger can be elicited by not eating. Soon food intake will be regulated by the infant's emotional instead of physiological needs.

This developmental deficit, the lack of somatopsychological differentiation, underlies the basis of infantile as well as the adolescent anorexia nervosa. In order to understand the difficulties in this developmental process, it is important to examine the contribution of the infant's temperament, the mother's conflicts and the father's involvement or lack of engagement with the mother and the infant.

TREATMENT

The focus of treatment lies in improving communication between parents and infant in order to facilitate the development of somatopsychological differentiation as part of the separation and individuation process of the infant. A two-step therapeutic approach has proven useful in determining two major groups of mothers and infants with infantile anorexia nervosa.

The first step involves a cognitive behavioral intervention aimed at helping the parents understand and promote the development of their infant's somatopsychological differentiation. The therapist begins the intervention by meeting with both parents and explaining the developmental conflict of their infant around autonomy and dependency and expression of this conflict through food refusal:

> The infant has learned to assert his autonomy by refusing to eat. This has generated parental anxiety about the infant's food intake and physical growth and resulted in increased efforts to enhance food intake. Although their coaxing, cajoling, playing distracting games, or force-feeding has not been successful in increasing the infant's food intake, the parents' abundant attention around the infant's food refusal has certainly encouraged the infant's emotional appetite. The food refusal has worked for the infant in two ways: allowing him to assert his autonomy by refusing to eat while concurrently meeting his need for attention. This has given the infant a sense of control that has perpetuated the pattern. The infant's emotional hunger for attention has outweighed his physiological hunger for food; he is failing to develop somatopsychological differentiation, the ability to separate physiological from emotional need.

Following this explanation of the infant's developmental conflicts, the parents are provided with behavioral techniques aimed at allowing the infant more autonomy during feeding and setting limits on inappropriate, maladaptive behaviors at the same time. They are given some general "food rules": to facilitate self-feeding by offering fingerfood, a second spoon, or a little dish with food while feeding the infant; to feed the infant at regular times and not to offer milk and snacks between these regular meal and snack times in order to allow the infant to experience hunger; to limit mealtimes to 30 minutes and to terminate the meal earlier if the infant refuses to eat, throws food, or eating utensils in anger or to provoke the parents, or if the infant plays with the food without eating. In order to facilitate somatopsychological differentiation, to help the infant distinguish physiological hunger for food from emotional hunger for attention, the parents are encouraged to separate mealtimes from playtimes. They are asked to deal with the infant's food intake in a neutral manner, neither playing games to distract the infant in order to sneak a bite into the infant's mouth nor clapping their hands and making a big production for every mouthful the infant swallows. Parents also are requested to withhold expressions of disapproval and frustration if the infant eats little or nothing. They are reassured that experiencing hunger is the only means of inducing the infant to eat. In this way, the infant's attention can be focused on his inner state of hunger or satiety rather than on his interactions with the parents. Parents are encouraged to introduce a playtime after the meal in order to provide the attention they previously showered on the infant in their efforts to induce him to eat.

Parents who are able to support one another can apply this approach and usually, within a few days or weeks, they succeed in changing the infant's eating pattern. However, parents in conflict with one another whose relationship is fraught with control issues, frequently have difficulty joining together in treatment. This usually becomes evident in their inability to attend appointments together. The mother is usually most distressed by the infant's food refusal and frequently reports that the father feels "it is all her fault." These mothers are so overwhelmed with guilt and self-doubt that any suggestion of handling the infant in a different manner, even if couched in the most careful developmental terms, is frequently interpreted as criticism and experienced as confirmation that they are "bad" mothers. The opening door for these mothers can be in the question, "Do you feel comfortable with these new food rules?" or after the mother has tried to change her handling of the infant according to the food rules, "What parts of these food rules are hard for you to deal with?" These questions allow the mother to describe her problems with limit setting and saying "no" to her infant. In exploring the mother's conflicts in this area the second phase of treatment is introduced.

This second phase of treatment can involve individual psychotherapy for the mother in cases where the mother appears to struggle with unresolved conflicts over autonomy and control exacerbated by the infant's entering the developmental phase of separation and individuation. Treatment must put the ghosts to rest. The mother needs to feel that the therapist listens to her with empathy, without the critical attitude the mother perceived in her mother. As she experiences "mirroring" by the therapist, the mother's own capacity to mirror her infant begins to develop. As the therapist explores the mother's struggles for control and her sense of helplessness during her growing years in her battles with her own mother, the mother begins to draw parallels between her relationship with her own mother and her interactions with her infant.

She begins to understand that in her effort to be a "better" mother she has gone to the other extreme of being too permissive and indulgent; she will explore her suppressed rage that periodically erupted in the past and frightened her because she found herself acting "just like her mother." The therapist will help the mother to understand her anger and explore alternative modes of setting limits with her infant.

During this psychotherapeutic work, the mother's relationship with the infant's father assumes an important role. Frequently similar conflicts around control and dependency are evident. In some cases couple's therapy becomes a natural progression of the therapeutic work. In other situations the conflict is so intense that the parents engage in repeated separations and reunions without resolution of the underlying difficulties in their relationship.

CASE HISTORIES

Two cases representative of a mild and a more severe form of infantile anorexia nervosa are described:

Case 1

M., a 12-month-old Caucasian girl, was referred by her pediatrician for a psychiatric evaluation because of failure to thrive and feeding problems. The pediatric assessment had revealed a deceleration of growth beginning at nine months of age, with recent measurements of height and weight falling below the third percentiles for age. There was no organic illness to explain this growth failure.

M. was the second child of young middle-class, college-educated parents. The mother had experienced some bleeding during the fifth month of pregnancy when the diagnosis of placenta previa was made. This had led to increased anxiety about the infant's health for the rest of the pregnancy. M. had to be delivered by Caesarean section during the ninth month of pregnancy. She weighted 5 lbs. 7 oz. at birth, had a somewhat weak suck for the first few days but otherwise had been a healthy and delightful baby.

For the first six months of life M.'s development was age-appropriate and without any difficulties. The mother stayed at home to care for M. and her brother, who was three years older. The mother explained that this was very important to her because she had grown up with her own mother working after her father had deserted the family. She had experienced her own mother as unavailable and overwhelmed. M.'s mother and father had planned to provide a better childhood experience for their children. She breastfed M. and very much enjoyed the closeness with her baby during the first six months. At six months of age, on the suggestion of the pediatrician, the mother introduced baby foods, but felt that M. did not seem very interested. The mother noticed that if she entertained M. with toys or music she could slip food into M.'s mouth without the baby attending to the feeding. However, with time it became increasingly difficult to distract M. in order to induce her to eat. By nine months of age, M. would stubbornly refuse to open her mouth when mother attempted to feed her. As her motor development progressed M. would wiggle off her mother's lap and toddle away to play with toys instead of eating. The mother became increasingly anxious about M.'s poor food intake. She worked harder to distract M. in order to feed her but M. only became more resistant. By the time of the evaluation, the mother described spending one to two hours per meal attempting to feed M., even frequently putting her in the bath tub with watertoys to keep M. physically confined in order to get to her mouth. The mother admitted to great frustration because she had tried "everything" to pique M.'s interest in solid food, though without success. The mother also noted that M. would frequently ask for the breast; and at this point, M. was getting her nourishment primarily from the breast, with minimal oral intake of solid food.

The observation of mother and infant during 20 minutes of feeding and 10 minutes of play revealed the following interactional patterns: M. was a vivacious, tiny girl who seemed to take in the world around her with great interest and pleasure. The mother had brought a variety of toys, including a music box which she placed on the table to prepare for the feeding. The mother chose to feed M. with the baby sitting on her lap although a highchair was available. The mother turned on the music and sang and talked to M. while she attempted to feed her. M. took a bite and grabbed for the spoon, but the mother maintained her hold and filled the spoon with food. The mother appeared completely unaware that M. wanted to feed herself. When the mother tried to give M. the next spoonful, M. refused to open her mouth, wiggled off the mother's lap, and walked to the toys. Mother pleaded for M. to return, took a doll, and showed M. how to feed the doll. M.

appeared fascinated by this play. While M. was busy imitating her mother in feeding the doll the mother was able to slip another spoonful into M.'s mouth. When M. toddled away again, the mother followed her with the spoon attempting to catch her for another bite. M. thoroughly enjoyed this chase, giggled and squirmed when her mother caught her but refused to open her mouth. As she ran out of ideas for tricking M. into eating, the mother appeared increasingly saddened and frustrated although she maintained a good show for her infant.

The play that followed this feeding sequence revealed similar interactional patterns. The infant took the lead in their interactions, bringing the mother toys and the mother responded with interest and pleasure. However, when M. seemed absorbed in manipulating a toy box, the mother took some finger food from her purse and tried to slip it into M.'s mouth. These observations revealed that the mother appeared preoccupied with the task of getting food into the infant's mouth without having any awareness of M.'s drive for autonomy expressed during the feeding by grabbing the spoon and playing games with mother, representing both, M.'s need for attention and her drive for independence.

Both parents came for the interpretive session. While looking at the videotape of the feeding and play session described previously, the parents were able to recognize that M. acted out her developmental conflict between autonomy and dependency through food refusal. The mother was reinforced in her ability to engage with the infant in high-level symbolic play. After this reassurance, she seemed able to address her difficulty with limit setting. She described that during her childhood she and her siblings had been left largely to themselves, and that her mother would only interact and "yell" if things got out of control. The mother expressed her fear that she was becoming just like her mother. She was so exhausted by trying to feed M. that sometimes, her frustration was revealed by "yelling" at her infant. The mother was very grateful for being offered "the food rules," and to be given concrete suggestions on handling M. during mealtime. She readily changed her interactions with M., put her in a highchair, offered her a spoon and a little dish with babyfood and fingerfood, and was very pleased with the results. She felt so boosted in her new ability to deal with M. that she volunteered to use the same food rules with her son who was also a "picky" eater, although he had never pushed the mother as far as M. The father was very supportive of these new rules in the home and both parents felt comfortable in terminating treatment after five sessions.

Case 2

S., a 12-month-old Caucasian boy, was referred by his pediatrician for a psychiatric evaluation because of failure to thrive and feeding problems.

S. was the only child of his middle-aged parents. His father was a professional who worked as a consultant out of his home. His mother was college-educated but had never enjoyed her career as a working woman. She had looked forward to starting a family and had readily relinquished her career to stay home with S. Her pregnancy with S. and the delivery were uneventful and mother and infant went home from the hospital three days after birth. S. weighed 6 lbs. 9 oz. and had a strong suck. Mother decided to bottle feed him and feeding began without difficulties. However, S. turned into an irritable baby who was difficult to soothe and to settle down for feedings. At five months of age he developed an ear infection; he became febrile and lethargic and refused to eat or drink. The mother became very concerned that he might become dehydrated until finally she was able to get him to drink some water while he seemed asleep. After he recovered from the ear infection he resumed feeding, but a month later he developed his second ear infection and then became ill at least once a month. Each time he was ill he did not want to eat or drink. This behavior frequently persisted for days. Around nine months of age S. developed thrush and became very difficult to feed. The mother reported that she had introduced solid food at five months of age and that S. had started throwing temper tantrums during feedings as early as eight months of age. However, when he developed thrush, feeding became an absolute struggle. The mother reported that she "had tried everything," distracting him with toys and kitchen utensils, coaxing him, offering him all kinds of food, and at times force-feeding him when everything else seemed to fail and she had been terrified that he might become dehydrated.

The mother expressed relief over having the opportunity to get psychiatric help. She admitted in tears that a few days prior to the diagnostic assessment S. had been so obstinate and difficult that she put him in the crib for punishment and left the room to calm herself. However, S. had screamed loudly for ten minutes until she could not bear it any longer and returned to his room to remove him from his crib. He refused to be taken out and tightly held on to the crib railing while the mother tried to lift him up. In the process she lacerated the tip of one of his fingers. The mother cried out in the interview that at that moment she had wished to tear off his whole finger. She was terrified by her rage.

A diagnostic session of 20 minutes of feeding followed by 10 minutes of play revealed the following interactional patterns: While the mother was still busy preparing her own food, S. eagerly helped himself to a few bites from the dish the mother had put in front of him. The moment the mother sat down to eat and her attention was focused on him S. stopped eating. He watched his mother's every move and whenever she looked his way he dropped an eating utensil from the tray on his highchair. He would point to another dish or some other food his mother had kept out of his reach. She would give it to him and pick up whatever he had thrown down. S. banged the spoons and plates on the tray, threw the food on the floor in a deliberate way with his eyes focused on his mother as if saying "I dare you, Mother, what are you going to do now?" The mother appeared paralyzed. She would rise from her chair, pick up the objects S. had thrown, and offer him toys or other eating utensils in a mechanical fashion. Her affect was flat, she barely spoke to the baby. When she tried to feed him intermittently, S. would refuse to open his mouth or push her hand away. The mother appeared increasingly distressed as S. escalated his provocative behaviors. During the whole session he hardly ate a bite.

During the play that followed, S. ran around the room in a frantic fashion. He picked up some blocks, banged them on the wall and against the mirror, and constantly provoked his mother by doing things she did not want him to do. The mother sat on the floor in resignation. She had tried to get S. interested in building blocks with her or to explore the busy box, but S. ignored her, ran away, and put his finger on the electric outlet. She screamed out "No." S. looked startled for a moment but tried a second time. This time the mother abruptly removed him from the electric outlet. S. looked bewildered, cried a little but then resumed his frantic pace.

Both parents came for the interpretive session. The mother was unable to watch the videotape of the feeding and play session described previously. She was so distressed and frightened about S.'s food refusal that her pediatrician agreed to hospitalize S. the following day.

During the hospitalization S. had tubes inserted in both ears to prevent further ear infections. He was put on a feeding protocol that included a regimen of regular meals and snacks and no bottles between meals. He was fed by nurses to break the pattern of maladaptive behaviors he had developed with his mother and to neutralize the feeding situation in order to help him learn to eat according to his hunger sensations instead of his emotional needs. The mother stayed with S. in the hospital. She had great difficulty separating from S. for mealtimes and regularly handed in written complaints about the incompetence of the nursing staff. Eventually, when she could spend time with the therapist while S. was being fed by the nurses, the mother was able to handle the situation more effectively. S. engaged in provocative behaviors during feedings with the nursing staff and quickly determined those nurses he could control. He responded to kind but firm limit setting but his actual eating behavior increased only slowly; his poor caloric intake was supplemented through nightly nasogastric tube feedings with the help of a feeding pump. S. gained weight gradually, his eating improved slowly. After two weeks his mother resumed his feedings according to the new food rules. S. was discharged after three weeks in the hospital. He was a much more engaging and happy little boy.

Mother and S. continued in psychotherapy. Mother revealed that she had been in psychoanalysis for eight years, and that her analyst had forewarned her during termination that her conflictual feelings toward her mother might resume when she had her own children. Mother described her childhood as an ongoing battle with her mother whom she experienced as intrusive, controlling, and inconsistent. Her mother had told her spitefully that S. was going to make her feel what she (the mother's mother) had experienced when she would not eat as a child. The mother recalled in pain how "her mother had blocked out the sun of her childhood" and she expressed her fear that she was going to do the same to S. At times it was difficult for the mother to separate her angry feelings toward her mother from her feelings toward S. and she wondered out loud whether the conflict with S. would continue forever in the same way as her conflict with her mother had never stopped. During these sessions S. would intently watch his mother and at times cry when she appeared to be in pain. At home the feedings seemed to reflect the emotional seesaw between mother and infant.

The mother did not want to involve the father in the treatment and initially did not allow the father to feed S. She decided that the father's constant presence in the house was too intrusive and she arranged with him to work out of an office away from home. After this move she allowed the father to take over the breakfast feeding for S. In the treatment she explored her disappointment in her marriage and how S. had displaced her husband. Both she and her husband felt increasingly exhausted because there was no more life beyond taking care of S.

Gradually, she allowed the therapist to address her own needs. As she became more confident in her ability to mother S., the mother could see that she had needs that her child could not fulfill. She became more open to involving her husband with S. and introduced dinners together for all three of them. During this time S. blossomed, his speech and his play developed dramatically, and his affect brightened. When he was 22 months old S. engaged in tender, affectionate play with his mother. He would hug his mother for long periods of time while she was talking to the therapist. There was no more frantic running around. Mealtimes became more routine and mother reported that she very much enjoyed their play time afterwards.

CONCLUSION

Infantile anorexia nervosa is an eating disorder characterized by food refusal and failure to thrive that manifests during the early phase of separation and individuation. The onset is usually between six months and three years, most commonly around nine months of age. The infant refuses to eat in an attempt to achieve a degree of autonomy and control with regard to the mother, a maneuver that serves to involve the mother more deeply in the infant's eating behavior. The mothers are controlling in their interactions with their infants, miss and override the infant's cues, and seem unable to recognize the infant's attempts at self-feeding. Mother and infant appear to be out of step with one another in their interactions, leading both to experience increasing levels of frustration and distress. Because of the mother's inconsistent and noncontingent responses, the infant fails to develop somatopsychological differentiation, the ability to differentiate physiological sensations, such as hunger and satiety, from emotional feelings, such as need for affection or anger and frustration. As infant and mother become embroiled in a battle of wills over food intake, the infant's feeding becomes more directed by his emotional rather than his physiological needs.

Several factors appear to contribute to the development of this eating disorder. The infants appear to have a strong-willed temperament, amazing persistence, and remarkable sensitivity, enabling them to read the mother's cues and to understand cause and effect.

The mothers frequently struggle with unresolved conflicts around autonomy and control stemming from their relationship with their own mothers. These "ghosts from their nursery" become activated when their infants enter the developmental phase of separation and individuation, when infants become more expressive of their own desires and when mothers must balance between setting limits and fostering autonomy.

The father's psychopathology and involvement with the mother and the infant appear to be important variables that can determine the severity of the separation difficulties and eating disorder of the infant.

Treatment must consider all these factors. The focus of treatment lies in improving communication between parents and infant to facilitate the development of somatopsychological differentiation as part of the infant's process of separation and individuation.

The first intervention is aimed at helping the parents understand and promote this developmental process. In a cognitive-behavioral approach, the therapist provides the parents with explanations of the infant's behavior and suggests ways to structure mealtimes in order to shape the infant's behavior differently.

Parents whose conflictual relationship interferes with this process and mothers who struggle with unresolved control and dependency issues require couple's therapy or individual psychotherapy to address these conflicts as they continue to intrude in the relationship with their infant.

References

Bruch, H. (1973), *Eating Disorders, Obesity and Anorexia Nervosa and the Person Within*, Basic Books, New York.

Chatoor, I., and Egan, J. (1983), Nonorganic failure to thrive and dwarfism due to food refusal: A separation disorder, *J. Acad. Child Psychiatry, 22*, 294–301.

Chatoor, I., and Egan, J. (1987), Etiology and diagnosis of failure to thrive and growth disorders in infants and children, in J. Noshpitz

(Ed.), *Basic Handbook in Child Psychiatry*, Vol. V, Basic Books, New York, pp. 272–279.

Chatoor, I., and Egan, J. (1987), Treatment of failure to thrive and growth disorders in infants and children, in J. Noshpitz (Ed.), *Basic Handbook in Child Psychiatry*, Vol. V, Basic Books, New York, pp. 421–425.

Chatoor, I., Schaefer, S., Dickson, L., and Egan, J. (1984a), Nonorganic failure to thrive: A developmental perspective, *Pediatr. Ann., 13*, 829–843.

Chatoor, I., Schaefer, S., Dickson, L., Egan, J., Conners, C. K., and Leong, N. C. (1984b), Pediatric assessment of nonorganic failure to thrive, *Pediatr. Ann., 13*, 844–850.

Chatoor, I., Dickson, L., Schaefer, S., and Egan, J. (1985a), A developmental classification of feeding disorders associated with failure to thrive: Diagnosis and treatment, in D. Drotar (Ed.), *New Directions in Failure to Thrive: Research and Clinical Practice*, Plenum, New York, pp. 235–258.

Chatoor, I., Getson, P., Himmelberg, P., Dickson, L., Schaefer, S., Egan, J., and Einhorn, A. (1985b), Observational scales for infants and mothers during feeding and play (Abstract), *Proceedings of the 32nd Annual Meeting of the Academy of Child Psychiatry*, San Antonio, Texas, p. 36.

Chatoor, I., Egan, J., Getson, P., Menvielle, E., and O'Donnell, R. (1988), Mother–infant interactions in infantile anorexia nervosa, *J. Am. Acad. Child Adolescent Psychiat., 27*, 535–540.

Egan, J., Chatoor, I., and Rosen, G. (1980), Nonorganic failure to thrive: Pathogenesis and classification, *Clinical Proceedings, Children's Hospital National Medical Center, 36*, 173–182.

Fraiberg, S., Adelson, E., and Shapiro, V. (1975), Ghosts in the nursery, *J. Acad. Child Psychiatry, 14*, 387–421.

Freud, A. (1946), The psychoanalytic study of infantile feeding disturbances, *Psychoanal. Study Child, 2*, 119–132.

Greenspan, S. I., and Lourie, R. S. (1981), Developmental structuralist approach to classification of adaptive and pathologic personality organizations: Infancy and early childhood, *Am. J. Psychiatry, 138*, 725–735.

Greenspan, S. I., and Lieberman, A. F. (1981), Infants, mothers and their interaction: A quantitative clinical approach to developmental assessment, in S. I. Greenspan, and G. H. Pollock (Eds.), *The Course of Life, Vol. I. Infancy and Early Childhood*, U.S. Government Printing Office, Washington, D.C., pp. 271–312.

Mahler, M. S., Pine, F., and Berman, A. (1975), *The Psychological Birth of the Human Infant*, Basic Books, New York.

Rizzuto, A. M., Peterson, R. K., and Reed, M. (1981), The pathological sense of self in anorexia nervosa, *Psychiatric Clinics of North America, 4*, 471–487.

Palazzoli, M. (1974), *Self-Starvation*, Jason Aronson, Northvale, New Jersey.

Winnicott, D. M. (1971), *Playing and Reality*, Basic Books, New York.

Woolston, J. (1985), Diagnostic classification: The current challenge in failure to thrive Research, in D. Drotar (Ed.), *Research and Clinical Practice*, Plenum, New York, pp. 225–233.

Children's Hospital National Medical Center
111 Michigan Avenue, N.W.
Washington, D.C. 20010

SEXUALITY, PREGNANCY, AND PARENTING IN ANOREXIA NERVOSA

S. LOUIS MOGUL, M.D.

This paper brings together disparate ideas that have interested me in trying to understand the complicated illness that is anorexia nervosa. It presents questions, contradictions, and paradoxes. Even its general clinical usefulness is questionable, though the major part is a presentation of details of an interesting psychoanalysis of a woman whose first, aborted, pregnancy marked the start of anorexia nervosa and whose second, desired, pregnancy marked the recovery from anorexia and the beginning of a happy family.

Anorexia nervosa is a disease that turns its victims against nature and, even, against life itself. Along with the repudiation of nutritional needs, which poses a threat to individual survival, goes a repudiation of sexuality in terms of psychological interest and physiological functioning, resulting in major interference with reproduction. For females, who make up 90-95% of anorectics, there is regression to prepubertal or pubertal levels of hormones (Katz et al., 1978), manifested in amenorrhea. Studies of male anorectics show a similar loss of sexual interest and potency (Crisp and Burns, 1983) and regression also to prepubertal or pubertal hormonal levels (Crisp et al., 1982; Beumont et al., 1972).

There have recently been some papers taking issue with the claim that anorexia nervosa interferes with normal sexual attitudes, summarized in the polemical review of Scott (1987) who concludes, "there is little evidence for many widely held beliefs concerning psychosexual factors within eating-disordered patients" (p. 199). He cites, in particular, studies of Buvat-Herbaut et al. (1983) and Beumont et al. (1981) and states, "In sum, there appears to be nothing to particularly substantiate a suggestion of oddities within the sexual outlook or behavior among anorectics" (p. 204). Scott dismisses as "anecdotal" the wide clinical experience (Bruch, 1973; Crisp, 1980; Dally and Sargent, 1966; Sours, 1980; Thomas, 1967; among many others) that is inconsistent with his

S. Louis Mogul is an Assistant Clinical Professor, Department of Psychiatry, Harvard Medical School.

view, even though this view is based on reports with major methodological problems. Buvat-Herbaut et al. refer to their patients as having anorexia nervosa but do not make a distinction between anorexia nervosa and bulimia, a distinction that is crucial for the issue of sexuality. Their reliance entirely on a questionnaire for their data does not deal with anorectics' pronounced tendency to speak in terms of conventional norms, which are contradicted by their actual behavior. Beumont et al. (1981) and Abraham and Beumont (1982) do in fact distinguish between restricter anorectics and bulimics and their study strongly confirms the picture of the restricter anorectics, in contrast to bulimics, as ascetic and childlike in asexual and antisexual attitudes and behavior.

By anorexia nervosa I refer, in accord with DSM-III-R (1987), to that more ascetic disorder involving a distorted body image of being too fat, in which weight loss and extreme thinness are pursued mainly by dietary restriction and exercise, in contrast to bulimia nervosa where there are binges and weight control (not necessarily loss to the point of extreme thinness) mainly by vomiting, purging, and/or diuresing. In the latter, there is not only indulgence in eating binges, but, not infrequently, in smoking, drinking, and sexual activity. It is certainly true that there are many mixed cases, with sequential, cyclical, or overlapping clinical states, indicative of some common etiological factors. Still, this definitional distinction is important as the physiology and the psychology of the two clear-cut states are different and this difference is highly relevant for the issues of this paper, namely, sexuality (including sexual identity), pregnancy, and parenting in women with anorexia nervosa.

I

These issues present some challenging paradoxes. Anorexia nervosa is a peculiarly human disease. Yet, there are a large number of animal anorexias in various species, ranging from mollusks through fish, reptiles, and birds, to both sea and land mammals, reviewed in a very interesting paper by Mrosovsky and Sherry (1980), from which I take the following material:

> There are times when animals eat very little and lose weight, even when food is present. In many species this occurs when the animal is engaged in other important activities that compete with feeding. For example, bull

seals go without feeding for several weeks while they defend their territory and harem; to feed would entail their going into the water and leaving their territory unprotected. Fasting also occurs in association with incubation, migration, molting and hibernation, even though food is sometimes readily available. Such fasting can be distinguished from the outset from the fasting of sick animals because it occurs regularly, at specific stages of the life cycle.

. . . We argue that eating very little, even when plentiful food is provided, reflects an adaptation to predictable periods when food is unavailable in nature, either because it is in short supply, or because an activity of greater importance, which would be disturbed by feeding, is going on. (p. 837)

With the exception of molting, and to some extent hibernation, all of these other "activities of greater importance" are more or less directly in the service of reproduction. Even hibernation is in the service of having the young not born at a time of scarcity of food. In other instances, the connection with reproduction is very direct. For the mouth-breeding cichlids, the female of which incubates the eggs in their mouths, there is incompatibility between feeding and breeding and they tend to reject food during this time. In every species, it is only the directly involved gender that becomes anorectic and loses weight. In animals such as seals and deer, in which defense of territory and harem is important, it is only the male who reduces eating. Stags in captivity provided plentiful food still reduce eating and lose weight in the rutting season. The junglefowl hen reduces food intake by 80% during the 20 days of incubation and loses 10–20% of her body weight. The male, who has no part in this and does not provide food for the hen, does not lose weight. Both male and female emperor penguins fast while walking 40–50 days to their breeding sites. The female then goes to sea and the male assumes the incubation duty for the next 62–64 days while hatching. At this time, he will have lost 40% of his body weight. In contrast to emperor penguins, both male and female king penguins undergo courtship fasts and then have alternating incubating fasts, each gender losing 10–20% of its weight.

Mrosovsky and Sherry provide convincing evidence that these animal anorexias are regulated by a progressive lowering of the set point for body fat, thus avoiding the tension of hunger that would be there if body fat fell far below the operating set point. The raising and lowering of this set point is the basis of an internally regulated cycle of major weight loss and gain that is highly adaptive and operates without causing apparent distress.

Many people in our affluent society spend much effort to lose weight; few succeed over long periods and many wish they had a "touch" of anorexia to help in their struggle. The above-cited animal data led me to speculate whether some individuals who become anorectic are in fact initiating a progressive lowering of the set point for body fat without control over termination. This might be reflected on the psychological level in the distorted body image of being too fat, which also progressively descends. There is no question that people who become anorectic wish to lose weight and that powerful current cultural and family values about body size and shape are operative, giving rise to growing numbers of sufferers from this disease, but there is very much the question about why some individuals are able to be so effective at losing weight by exercise and fasting alone with more or less obvious distress, without resorting to vomiting, purging, or diuresing.

Often important life issues seem involved in precipitating anorexia nervosa, especially developmental issues in the sexual and reproductive areas. Some few individuals describe the onset of anorexia as the result of what seems like an ordinary plan to lose weight. In either case, the anorexia, like a pact with the devil, takes on a directed force of its own that is often experienced as exhilarating in the beginning, but eventually, if it continues, drags its victim down to hell.

The animal anorexias are vitally necessary for individual survival in some species and for mating and reproduction in many others, and are carefully regulated by biological mechanisms. They are, thus, relatively obligatory and near universal in those species and genders where they occur. (Interestingly, where individual survival is too much threatened, anorexia in the service of reproduction may be abandoned. For example, the emperor penguin will leave his egg prematurely if weight falls below the point where fat reserves are exhausted and protein catabolism increases.) Can it be that some few human individuals who wish to lose weight for whatever reason—cosmetic, competition in self-control or self-assertion; family or societal mores; ascetic defenses against growing up, especially sexually, or even against primitive unconscious wishes—trigger some comparable biologic mechanism for progressive lowering the set point for fat that dampens or shuts down many vital activities? If any of this does operate in anorexia nervosa, its maladaptive nature is exemplified in the turning on of this potentially destructive force without the reliable capacity to turn it off.

II

Anorexia nervosa has had a long and checkered career within psychoanalysis, starting, unidentified as such, with Freud's Rat Man case (1909/1965), the subject of which left the table "before the pudding came round" and certainly exercised frantically to "make himself slimmer" (p. 188). Freud responded to this as one more obsession and focused his attention on the significance of the unconscious metaphorical word play. ("Dick," the English name of his rival in love vs. "dick," the German word for fat.)

Starting in the 1940s, analysts paid attention to anorexia nervosa as a disease entity in which conflicts around orality and primitive aspects of female sexuality were the focus (Kaufman and Heiman, 1964). The view of not eating, vomiting, and weight loss with amenorrhea as a defense against unconscious phantasies of oral impregnation was elevated to the role of a specific determinant. Indeed, some patients, especially unsophisticated ones, do report such phantasies or behave in ways consistent with them. Classical psychoanalytic treatment, however, particularly in its focus on primitive drives, has proven either unacceptable to, beyond the capacity of, or, in any event, ineffective for most anorectics.

In recent years, the drive-centered view of early analytic workers has been rather thoroughly discredited and has even become the whipping post of many writers. Bruch (1973) led the way to a more fruitful view that distortions of early development in which parents, especially mothers, interfere with the growth of a separate, effective, worthwhile sense of self are determining for the future of anorexia nervosa. Even with this valuable perspective providing better understanding of the disorder and more effective interventions, treatment of anorexia nervosa using any and all of the contemporary modalities continues to be long and difficult, and often has a disappointing outcome.

This calls for dynamic psychotherapists and psychoanalysts to (1) be open to relevant input from biology, sociology, and family study; (2) refine understanding of early developmental sources; and (3) consider later, more contemporary issues in the lives of those who become anorectic. In this latter connection, despite considerable controversy, I am impressed with the importance in precipitating anorexia of becoming a grown woman, including the areas of sexuality, love relationships, procreation, feminine identity, as well as autonomy and career achievement.

III

Severe anorexia nervosa precludes pregnancy. Not only is there lack of sexual desire and activity but the physiological basis of fertility is shut down. On the other hand, anorexia nervosa not uncommonly has its onset with pregnancy in post-adolescents and some such pregnancies go to term despite the illness. Also, women with not so severe cases, or in the recovery phase in more severe cases, may become pregnant even while still amenorrheic, and some of these pregnancies may come to term, especially if there is some weight gain during its course. The risks to the fetus and mother are increased in such pregnancies and it is generally recommended that anorectics wait until recovery is well established before becoming pregnant (Garfinkel and Garner, 1984).

With all the physiological and psychological forces arraigned against reproduction in women with anorexia, it is amazing and ironic that some anorectic women want to have children and, in fact, do so. Namir et al. (1986) recently reported on six cases of restricter anorectics who mostly wanted children and used the need to nourish the "baby" as a means of allowing themselves to gain weight during the pregnancies. They all had healthy babies, but returned to more severe anorectic thinking and behavior within six weeks after delivery.

Stewart and Rankin (1988) reported on the outcome of 23 pregnancies in 18 women who were either restricter anorectics (4), bulimics (3), or in remission (11) at the time of conception. For those who were ill at conception, there was continuation of the eating disorder, less gain in weight, and more fetal complications, including two fetal deaths, and lower birth weights and Apgar scores in four of those who survived. In one year follow-up, all seven of those mothers who were ill at conception remained ill and only two of the eleven who were in remission at conception were ill. These authors also recommend waiting a year after recovery before becoming pregnant.

IV

Viewing parenthood as a powerful developmental challenge and opportunity, I have been interested in capitalizing on this when it has come up with some patients who become anorectic during pregnancies, not only to avoid repetition of harmful childhood experiences, but to take advantage of the opportunity for restructuring of important parts of the self for the benefit of the new parent as well as the child.

I have worked with two women in extensive psychotherapy and one in psychoanalysis who have sought to find in their own good parenting some restitution of deficits they experienced in being parented. All had antecedent family environments leading to internalized attitudes about eating and weight that can be seen in retrospect as anlages for anorexia nervosa, but none had had an overt eating disorder until her early 20s, and in each instance serious cases of anorexia nervosa appeared early in pregnancies. Each case has its own individual characteristics but there are a number of intriguing common features. The husbands of all three were generally competent and accomplished people, caring, tolerant, and nurturing of their wives, who transferred many dependencies onto them. To varying degrees, each patient described unhappy childhoods based mainly on difficult relationships with mothers who are painted as depressed, bitter, limited people (like the mothers in the study of Bemporad and Ratey (1985)) who were cold to these daughters and enormously controlling of their sense of separateness and autonomy, as pictured by Bruch (1973). Each of these women had experienced a tight bond with her mother and very much viewed the world through her mother's eyes without realizing these limits until she actually left the family home.

One of the psychotherapy patients spoke of growing up as a very naive youngster, trained by her parents to see her mother as the perfect standard of womanhood whose judgments and expectations of her children were not to be questioned. "My mother experienced me as an extension of herself. I rarely felt I was a separate person with ideas and feelings of my own. Not until I got married did I realize what an empty shell of a person she was, altogether obsessed with physical appearance and housekeeping, and how unacceptable to her was my growing beyond being a compliant, asexual child."

All three of these women complained of their mothers' lack of support of, and even hostility to, their finding any pride or pleasure in budding pubertal development, resulting in a deficient or profoundly ambivalent sense of feminine identity and serious concern about the kind of mothering they would be able to provide. The patients' mothers gave lip service to valuing education and career achievement for women, and were bitter at not having had this for themselves, but were, in fact, unsupporting or even condemning of their daughters' ambitions in this direction as disloyal. With the treatment, the children of each of these patients all eventually did well despite their mothers' misgivings. All of the women were delighted to discover, in contrast to their own mothers, that their narcissistic pleasure as mothers was enhanced by their children's separateness and, even, assertive independence.

The first of the psychotherapy patients was in the midst of a graduate program at a prestigious university, where she found gratifying academic success and a new sense of liberation from her family, when she became pregnant shortly after marrying. She very much wanted children but not at this point, knowing it would be a major interference with her studies. Abortion was not legal at the time, so she unhappily continued the pregnancy. She became alarmed at the prospect of gaining weight and developed severe anorexia nervosa with some recovery after the birth of her child. She became pregnant again a little more than one year later and again became severely ill with anorexia that continued for several years before she entered treatment.

The second psychotherapy patient was also in the midst of a successful professional education when she married, hoping to have a child soon. Her anorexia started with her pregnancy, when she, too, became appalled at the thought of becoming fat. The anorexia was eventually complicated by vomiting, a clinical condition that persisted despite treatment with several different therapists.

I shall present a much more detailed picture of a young woman who developed the typical symptoms of anorexia nervosa while pregnant in the course of her successful four-year psychoanalysis, focusing on her entering into anorexia and then leaving it behind.

All three women used their therapies for anorexia nervosa, with my active focusing on parenting as a second chance, to extract from their successful parenting and loving relationships with their children not only major restitution of childhood emotional deficits in varying ways, but also significant restructuring of their feminine identities and senses of themselves as separate and worthwhile parents and persons.

V

Ms. K.

Ms. K. was a 21-year-old college student, attractive, intelligent, and articulate, who sought psychotherapy for troubling obsessive fears that were a recurrence of symptoms she had suffered with

SEXUALITY, PREGNANCY, AND PARENTING 73

intensely in childhood. She had recently come to the Boston area to continue her education and was living with a man several years older with whom she was very much in love. Her happiness began to be marred as the relationship became closer and, alone in a strange city, she experienced increasing emotional dependence on him. She had obsessive thoughts of great harm befalling her lover when she was apart from him. She knew this was neurotic and was terrified that it would take almost complete possession of her as it did for years in childhood when she was tortured by such thoughts during separations from her parents, especially her mother.

She was the younger of the two children of a wealthy upper-class family from a midwest metropolitan area. She spoke of her mother as an insecure unhappy woman, cold and controlling with her, who impressed her stamp on family life. Her mother was unhappy that she had not accomplished more with her own life, but was so obsessed with proper appearance, especially of personal looks and thinness, that she did not follow through on undertakings, such as her interest in becoming a psychologist. Ms. K. had many complaints about her mother, the most direct being, "My mother made me completely dependent on her and then criticized and nailed me for it." The patient felt that she had organized her life around pleasing her mother and was the "good, responsible child and conscientious student who never caused trouble" in contrast to her older brother, who was the source of worries and had no real accomplishments. Yet her brother was favored and more warmly loved by the mother.

She remembered her father as much warmer in childhood and as a source of some joy to her, but he too was insecure and, as she grew up, she lost respect for him. She did not much value his being a successful businessman and community leader. At home, he was too much under her mother's domination, bumbling, and ineffective.

There was a quality of adolescent exaggeration in this critical, belittling picture of her family, but she persisted in it for a long time. She dealt with her parents as though there were a continuing danger of being sucked back into the family fold if she did not actively ward this off.

There were several sources of happiness in childhood: (1) the black cook, Cora, fat and warm, but with dignity, who was loved by all the family and who made the patient her favorite; (2) the family dogs; (3) her private life of music, reading, and imagination; and (4) playing with other children with whom she achieved the status of a tomboy.

Evenings when her parents would go out were the worst part of childhood. She would be obsessed with images of their being hurt or killed in an accident and afraid of dying herself. She would become unhappy and clinging in anticipation of their departure, arousing the ire, instead of sympathy, of her mother. Her parents brought her to a child analyst for treatment, but she found this objectionable, was quite resistent, and felt it was of little benefit.

In adolescence, she began to feel some detachment from her parents and growing independence. The opportunity for play as a tomboy, however, was shut off and she felt isolated from and contemptuous of the "shallow, materialistic teenage scene" around her. She felt that the only way to avoid being sucked back into the whirlpool of dependence and identification with her mother's hated way of life was to leave home. She spent high school years relatively happily at a boarding school where she made several congenial relationships, including those with two boys with whom she had friendships as well as romantic and erotic involvements.

She met her current lover in college where he was known as one of the brighter intellects and poets. She revered these qualities and also saw him as a kindred soul. By the time they moved to Boston, they had a firm commitment to each other that Ms. K. insisted was more meaningful and durable than a marriage. Her parents, who supported them financially, wanted them to get married, but she was adamantly opposed. "Marriages are meant to hold together lousy relationships like theirs. We don't need that kind of coercion. It's a matter of firm principle."

They lived as simple, frugal vegetarians, yet there was clearly plenty of money for tuitions, analysis, travel, car, and the basics of life. The patient did not acknowledge any recognition of generosity from her family; rather, there was anger at their using money to control her, however subtly.

Ms. K. had never had an eating disorder. She spoke of her mother's attitude about food, eating, and body weight as the paradigm of how she put her stamp on family life. Thinness was a guiding force in her mother's life, for herself and all her family. They were all thin and had contempt for anyone who was fat except for their cook. Ms. K. herself felt a visceral disgust at fatness as though it were contagious. Meals were regularly major family occasions and were prepared and presented with thought and care. They were healthy, low in calories, and modest in quantity. "My mother discovered nouvelle cuisine on her own." You could ask for seconds but the price was parental scorn. Sweets were the special object of opprobrium. Tempting desserts were often prepared, but served only on explicit request and "in such tiny portions it wasn't worth it." Her mother never ate desserts. In like manner, there was generally a small supply of cookies in the house, not to be enjoyed, but to teach how to resist temptation. During the patient's adolescence, her mother would buy clothes that were too tight for her, which she experienced as mother's way of saying, "You are too fat."

After the patient became frankly anorectic, her mother confessed to some of her private eating habits such as buying a whole fresh baked bread, smelling it all the way home and then nibbling at the crust when she longed to eat the whole loaf. The patient realized, in a sudden flash, that her mother was a chronic, stable anorectic who so fully accepted the anorectic ethos that she established many aspects of anorexia as the family norm.

In her psychotherapy, Ms. K. was guarded at first but formed a positive therapeutic relationship. She was pleased with the considerable symptom relief and became fascinated with the experience of sharing her inner, imaginative life with her therapist. She started out very leary of psychoanalysis, with the opinion that her parents' "analyses" had not made them better people or parents. She felt it particularly important for her not to form a dependent relationship with me and the idea of a transference relationship, which she was intellectually quite aware of, was abhorrent to her, as she feared it would undo the hard-won emotional separation from her parents. After a year of psychotherapy, she pressed to go ahead with a psychoanalysis, and we did.

She arrived for the first analytic session quite excited over an "amazing transference dream." She reported the dream as follows:

On my way to my appointment with you I see my father, who says he is on his way to his analysis (which was, in fact, long since finished) dressed in a brown tennis outfit. I thought, "What a dope he looks and acts like. I hope I don't have to acknowledge that he is my father."

In the waiting room I see three young women my age sitting there. I think, "This guy sees so many young women, but I am not jealous because I have the appointment and they will just have to wait." You open the door and I put my arm around you, claiming you. I know that I am supposed to lie down on the couch but I am quite afraid, especially when I see that there are a blanket and pillow and it looks like a bed. I lie down and you sit beside me and kiss me three or four times. I feel excited and think I'll faint. "Is this supposed to be happening? It must be right or else you wouldn't do it." You then invite me to join your family for dinner and I know we are not going to do anything wrong, i.e., sexual, and that I'll be included as one of the children in your family. That will be quite wonderful even though your wife seems severe.

I felt some image of a patient being held by a doctor, like a child held by a mother, and that is a movingly beautiful picture to me.

After the dream, my first thought was to apologize to Luke (her lover) for betraying him in the dream. Then I thought this is an important and valuable dream: (a) it's a warning to you of my vulnerability, which you must protect, and (b) it's a sign to me that you are more important to me now, despite my denial, and that I am tied to you for a long and important journey with great expectations. I do realize that my current contemptuous attitude about my father—my parents—can't be all there is, even if the image of my father as a dope, and you as wise, is how I feel.

In the first year of analysis, Ms. K. worked hard to master her fear that a positive relationship with her analyst would mean engulfment and loss of control. In fact, she developed an idealized transference in which she often pictured her analyst as a natural nourisher and a Freud-like figure in the form of a wise and demanding leader and teacher. She took up the analytic work actively; dreaming, associating, reconstructing her past, and exploring her phantasies, emotions, and behavior. The original symptoms no longer bothered her and she became involved in making a new, more mature life for herself.

She felt strong determination to make something significant of her life, in contrast to her mother, who had many dilettante-like interests but no real accomplishments. She was studying music history and theory in college and had been accepted into a graduate program in musicology. She decided, however, that she really wanted to study psychology, recognizing how much her fascination with her analysis and her identification with me, as well as rivalry with her mother, were operating and she applied for a highly competitive Ph.D. program in psychology.

In her personal life, she felt more and more free of neurosis. She undertook to enrich her life socially and culturally by exploring the world around her. Her sexual life improved and she began to enjoy cooking and eating, experiencing a liberation from the fear of enjoying food.

About six months into her analysis, she rather casually announced that she and Luke had decided to get married. She explained this radical change by saying that the entire family would be attending her grandfather's 80th birthday, and this would make a nice present for her grandfather. When I first tried to explore the significance of this change, she was uncharacteristically reticent. As the wedding approached, she experienced some uneasiness. She acknowledged fear that getting married would mean giving up choices and pose the danger of her becoming more in the position of her mother.

Altogether there was a shifting of perspective from that of a post-adolescent to that of a grown-up. Her husband-to-be began regular work and considered career plans more seriously than before. She talked with enthusiasm of her 3-year-old niece, Willa, whom she would encounter on visits to her parents' and experienced this as rekindling a desire to have children before too long. Much earlier she had thought of having 13 children.

In the midst of these positive experiences, several things of an untoward nature came together. She was rejected by the psychology doctoral program. Despite the fact that she had studied little psychology and that the program was well known to be highly competitive, she was angry and mortified.

She so much enjoyed cooking and eating now that she expanded to baking. She and Luke would bake delicious cookies on weekends and gorge themselves. Suddenly she discovered she had gained weight, about 10–12 pounds; her weight was up to a record 125 pounds. It was terribly important for her to regain control of her body. She could not eliminate her body's urge to eat but she could make her mind stronger than her body. She thought: "My God, how great it would be not to have to think about food, to be liberated from being hungry anymore." She began a program of running and exercise and determined to curb her appetite. In a little over a month she lost 14 pounds. I became concerned that she was expressing these anorectic wishes.

At this point, ten days before her wedding, she discovered she was pregnant. With this she felt overwhelmed. Things were happening too fast; her head was in a maelstrom and she felt she was losing control. Her first emotional response to learning she was pregnant was a moment of being ecstatic that she could have a real accomplishment that made her feel blessed. She was amazed at how physical the pregnancy was, from morning sickness to swollen breasts, and strange body sensations.

She then recognized that she did not want to have a baby now. They were not ready; she would lose control of her life and it would be a practical and emotional disaster, despite the part of her that had longed to have babies and still did. She had an abortion and was amazed that she felt more relief than depression when it was over. She was impressed with the power of her unconscious. For four years she had been consistently responsible with her diaphragm. She now recalled she had been clearly told that if her weight changed by more than 10 pounds she should be refitted and she forgot that. "Was I trying to make some compensation for the grad school rejection by giving myself a baby?"

Two days later, she left for her wedding, which, to her surprise, was both moving and enjoyable. She felt the humanness of her family as never before. Her parents were emotional and nervous and saw to it that everything was beautiful—flowers, music, and even the ceremony.

During this time, she was unmistakably swept up into the world of anorexia nervosa. When she first realized she had gained weight, she planned to lose what she had gained and return to her regular weight of 115 pounds. But she found her goal descending from 115 to 110, to 105; then she thought that if she could get to 100 pounds she would be freed of having to think of food and eating. What a liberation from the material world that would be! She would no longer have to feel guilty with every mouthful. "Hunger and fullness are only states of the mind. If I can subdue them, my mind can subdue the world."

Losing the first few pounds was hard work. After that, when she became pregnant, the experience took on a different quality. The food restriction took on a life of its own. Rather than the hard struggle not to eat and feeling deprived, she felt high—in a state of excitement, even exhilaration. "For so long I wanted to lose weight and could only with the greatest difficulty and, suddenly, I could and did with ease. In the beginning I hated not eating; now I am disgusted at eating. In the beginning the resistance to eating was from the outside; now that I am anorectic, it's an inside resistance. . . . I enjoy the anorexia even though I know it's insane. . . . I have this crazy idea—I want to be so skinny that I'll never again have to resist the urge to eat—even though I know that is impossible. . . . I am frightened of my idea—to eat and never gain, i.e., no connection between the two. Ugh, what an unpleasant, frightening thought. . . . I wish I were so thin that even my mother would encourage me to eat. . . ."

I quote another statement from this time: "I have a great need to be special. Mother wanted me to fit in at high school. I felt that would be like joining a herd of cattle and losing all individuality. In some way, all the suffering of anorexia is worth it to make me special."

In addition to running and exercising, she joined a ballet class. She never vomited, purged, or used diuretics. A month after her wedding, her weight was 100 pounds; two months later it was 95. She looked haggard and joyless. She was impressed that even her mother was concerned enough to direct her, "Tell your doctor I think you are too skinny." She reassured her parents, "Don't worry, he won't let anything happen to me."

She reported that her sexual appetite was "nonexistent." In addition, there was no erotic feelings, phantasies, or responses. She commented, "Since the pregnancy and abortion I am so particular about what goes inside me — into any part of my body. I don't want anything foreign inside me."

Her interest in people other than her analyst was diminishing to the vanishing point. "When you are totally absorbed with food and weight there is no room for anyone else. I can no longer enjoy even the thought of others, the talk of friends, great poetry, the music I loved." Apart from the thrill of losing weight, her only real pleasure at this time was to stand on an ocean beach and have the cold North-Atlantic waves pound her frail and always chilled body — this she described as "exhilarating."

Remarkably, she had an unflagging interest in her analysis. Many anorectic patients view the therapist as a threat to what is vital to them. She knew that I saw her anorexia as a disease dangerous to her body and soul and she was very thankful for this. She saw her analysis as the way to understand it and work her way out, finding her own way rather than having one imposed on her. She actively pursued her thoughts, associations, and dreams, as well as being open to my ideas in trying to understand what was happening to her.

In the beginning, her conscious idea in losing weight, as for many other anorectics, was to make herself more attractive, even though the only person who really mattered to her, her husband, found her very attractive until she became too skinny. I had picked up anorectic-like ideas when she first began to lose weight, just after she decided to get married without her clearly facing this significant transition. She firmly insisted that the anorexia really started in the couple of weeks that she was pregnant, before she consciously knew this. Despite an intense wish for children, she had a strong feeling of not being ready for this. She had first to consolidate something of her emotional maturation via her analysis and in visible accomplishment through her education to protect herself from the intense fear of becoming like her mother when she became a mother.

At the same time, her attachment to her analyst took on a newly intense idealization. There were phantasies of me as a wise and loving father teaching his children the lessons of nature. Several times she apologetically told me, "I need you to be perfect." She was enthusiastic about her discovery of Hilda Doolittle's *A Tribute to Freud* (1971) and identified herself with the loving analysand and her analyst with Freud's power to understand and call forth understanding in the patient. She informed me, to my surprise and dismay, that, some months before, she had noted a section of books on eating disorders on my book shelves and that the volumes on anorexia had been changed around several times, indicating my interest in the subject. (My dismay was from the concern that her wish to interest me had contributed to her involvement in this grave disease.)

There was also the worrisome fact that my four-week summer vacation was coming soon. She had felt pained at being left with previous departures, but she was much more afraid this time and, at first, tried not to think of it. She remembered that she had "forgot" to attend the final session of her childhood therapy when she was eleven and now realized this was to avoid the pain of goodbye. She saw the current situation of her powerful attachment to me as an opportunity to free herself on a fundamental level from being reduced to helpless, frightened dependence as in previous attachments and that anorexia nervosa, with its antinomous aspects, was a necessary part of this struggle that would require all her strength. On the one hand, anorexia gave her a sense of specialness as though she had the ability to fly, but in reality it made her feel like a pathetically sick child. She saw the coming separation as a milestone in her personal growth, calling for true understanding and mastery of old conflicts and maladaptive resolutions.

I informed her that if her weight went below 90 pounds she would need to be hospitalized and made practical arrangements for this, if necessary, during my vacation. I was quite worried about her as we separated. She expressed confidence that she would be able to avoid hospitalization: (1) because she was looking forward to starting a graduate program in musicology, and (2) knowing that she would not let anything interfere with her analysis. Her last comment before we parted was, "Last night, in the midst of all this dryness, I wept at the thought of your leaving. I can't bear starving myself into a state of not feeling."

When we met again four weeks later, she was very thin but in good spirits. Her weight had dropped to 90.5 by mid-vacation, but, since then, had started to go up and now was 93. She missed me painfully but was not obsessed, as she feared, with thoughts of my destruction. Instead, she had images of dialogues with me, giving her a sense that some valuable part of the analysis was with her and in her control.

She was surprised and pleased that the vacation month spent with her parents went well. She did not like many aspects of her mother, but felt some distance from this and did not feel them as contagious. She appreciated her mother's new interest in nurturing without controlling. Best of all, her niece was there in the grandparents' care and she saw how loving her father was with the child, reminding her of this aspect of her own childhood. Also, she and Luke had a wonderful time playing and being with the girl, who responded very positively to them, making her feel she could be a good mother and giving her a less conflicted, concrete image of parenthood. She felt happy to be starting graduate school, anticipating this would motivate her to invest in real achievement.

The night before returning to analysis, she had another "powerful transference dream" in which she was coming for her appointment with me. She was bringing her two sons, Isaac, aged 5 and Jacob, 3, to present to me for the first time. I respond, "How beautiful they are," confirming her sense of pride in them. Her association to their names pointed to their redeeming and fruitful roles. The summer encounter with her niece and this dream reestablished clearly that the core of her creative mission was to parent healthy, happy children.

She continued to be anorectic for the next year but the direction was changing. Her weight very slowly increased. Her desire for food returned and it again took effort to resist the urge to eat. Preoccupation with food continued to interfere with her involvement with people but she began to resist this more and more. The first major return of a lost function was the ability to read, study, and think. She found pleasure in studying music and thought of this as making up for the hurt and deprivation of the psychology rejection. She found special pleasure in studying medieval music;

even most musically educated people did not know the fine points of this esoteric area of the art.

As we came to the anniversary of the "momentous events" of the previous year leading to her pregnancy and anorexia, she actively reviewed what had happened with new understanding. She acknowledged that choosing to get married involved forcing grown up responsibility on her and Luke about which she had felt ambivalent. She feared Luke's going to work would endanger his special gifts as a philosopher-poet as he would be lost in a world of working ants. In addition to the narcissistic blow from the psychology rejection, she now saw this as shutting her off from specifically surpassing her mother, whose unrealized ideal was to be a psychologist.

As we approached the next summer break, she entered her hour after a long weekend in a state of agitation.

I felt the need, while away, to force myself to have a powerful insight that would push me beyond this anorectic morass, this morbid fear of eating, so that I can grow physically and emotionally and give up clinging to this little girl way of life. I had such an insight and, as I was arriving at your house, I had the phantasy that I tell you this wonderful insight and you pull out a gun and shoot me in the head. It's so real I am still shaking. We were visiting my parents and my niece was there as usual. As I watched Luke be with Willa with great skill, warmth, and love, bringing out the best in her, I thought, "Her gain is not his loss and they each clearly know this." This is the opposite of how it was with my parents and me. As I heard my father, who loves Willa very much, refer to her as "my little girl," I cringed remembering that that was just what he used to say to me and I felt compelled to stay his little girl to retain his love, and still do. That night I had a dream. Father and I are sitting at the kitchen table, he in pajamas and I in a nightgown, sneaking a snack together while Mother is up in the bedroom. My father was drinking whiskey (which he never does) and getting drunk. He started to pour another glass and I put my hand on his to try to stop him. He then picked me up to take me to the bathroom, saying he had to pee. I was becoming alarmed. He then exposed his erect penis and rubbed it against me. I screamed and ran to get Mother. She angrily accused me of seducing him. I pleaded with her and her response was, "I know he isn't that sexually capable by himself." I felt my heart sink; there was nowhere to turn. This is horrible, really horrible. I was startled by the directness of the dream. No disguises. I can't grow up. I have to stay Father's little girl to retain his love. If Mother sees my maturing femininity as a threat to her own, she is filled with jealousy and attacks me as a dangerous rival, so I have to retreat. Well, this is my insight (spoken with trembling voice). I guess it's not so great after all.

I ask why she undoes her accomplishment. Why so fearful of my response? "You will be like my mother. Insights are yours. If I claim them, you will be jealous and shoot me," she answers.

"You have to stay a little girl for Father's favor, unwomanly for Mother's, and anorectic to be my interesting and compliant patient," I comment.

Excitedly, she says, "Yes, yes. Last year, without realizing it, I was forcing you to continue to be available to me even on vacation by being so worrisomely anorectic. Thank God, I am beyond that now."

When we met again after the vacation she had the grave news that Cora, the much loved cook, was dying of cancer and, in fact, she did die a month later. She was very grieved at the loss of this wonderfully unambivalent relationship. Her greatest pain was "Cora will never know my children and give them the love she gave me and evoked in me." After this she began a real push to gain weight and three months later her periods returned.

She found herself paying a lot of attention to children she encountered. When she met the young daughter of one of her professors, she thought, "I know what I want." She read about pregnancy and babies, and phantasies of a baby filled her with pleasure. "To be pregnant will put the finishing touches on the recovery from anorexia. I'll have to eat for the baby. When I was pregnant before, I knew I couldn't have a baby. It's different now." She began actually to enjoy eating and felt confidence in not losing control and binging.

She celebrated getting over anorexia by removing her I.U.D. Her sexual appetite came back and lovemaking was more fulfilling than ever as they connected it with the wish to conceive. After this, each period was a disappointment. She had always liked the flowering plants in my office, especially some flowering maples, which blossomed profusely. She reported she had been trying to raise some of these plants without success and feared this to be a sign of her not being gifted at propagation. I then learned that she was starting with seeds, whereas I propagated mine from cuttings. To dispel her idealized view of my magical power, I explained this. She later told me that her cuttings thrived and blossomed and she reported on their progeny in follow-up notes.

After years of resentment at the feeling that her father held onto her by making her dependent for money, she screwed up her courage and confronted her father with her wish to be recognized as a responsible adult and to be given direct control of her trusts. He not only promptly did this but asked her to be executrix and trustee for his will and trust, as she was clearly the most sensible and mature one in the family.

For the first time she brought up the thought of ending her analysis. "No matter what happens here, I am never going to have a happy childhood for myself. With Cora's death I realized that you never fully appreciate a relationship without an ending." Even though she felt superstitiously reluctant to think of planning a termination before she was pregnant, we did make the tentative plan to end in another year.

About half a year later, she found she was pregnant and was very relieved and genuinely happy. She felt her life as a grown woman with a family was coming into place. The pregnancy went smoothly and was, in fact, the most gratifying experience of her life. The feared return of anorexia nervosa did not at all materialize; instead, she felt more confidently free of concerns about food and weight than ever. Misgivings came up mainly in dreams such as the following: "After washing my hair, I am setting it with strips of paper impregnated with my father's semen. I am suddenly alarmed at the thought, 'This could make me pregnant.' Then I realize I am already pregnant with my husband and I feel great relief." She recalled her wish for 13 children when she was 6 years old and wondered whether she had had such strange ideas in her childish imagination. She also recalled how such wishes increased the barrier between her and her mother.

She embraced her pregnancy; she was always aware of it. "It's a physical satisfaction; I am never alone. My mother hated all of her pregnancies. I used to have the superstitious fear that if I bragged about being pregnant or my children I'd be struck down, Niobe-like. I have broken out of a family doom."

Three months before the baby was born we ended the analysis. "What an enormous relief that I can feel terribly sad at losing you without panic or fear of harm or death to you, me, or my baby. I think of the young woman who will replace me and I feel a surge of envy. But, then, I remember I don't need you so much anymore and hope she will get help, too. It's very bittersweet to leave. Analysis is like gardening. When a particular growing season is over there is no going back." I found out at this time that she had kept a journal of her analysis. "With this journal, I can keep a clear vision in my imagination of that room where you and I met and grew to know each other."

After an arduous labor, she gave birth to a healthy girl and felt happy and satisfied. With this she interrupted her musicology program without major regrets, even though having access to it had been so meaningful and she had worked hard at it, gaining recognition from others and an inner sense of achievement. To be a mother was now all she could think of and it seemed amply fulfilling. After three months, she brought in her daughter for me to meet. The baby was lively and winning; the mother was loving, proud, and clearly competent.

We met at monthly intervals for the next nine months, giving me an opportunity to follow her experience of being a mother. I report a few quotes:

> I have a baby, a house, and a dog. I am in love with my husband and enjoy making love. . . . Here I am, a housewife; but I know what I am doing. I'll ask for an academic extension; eventually I'll finish my degree work.
>
> . . . I am in love with my daughter more passionately than I ever imagined it possible to be. It's sad that when I was a baby girl I was not so loved by my mother. I can't believe that, but mother acknowledges it. She says she loves me more now than when I was little. . . . My mother didn't get that love from her mother and didn't have it to give to me. I have it with my girl and get it back through mothering her. . . . It was unfair to have to grow up feeling unlovable and that the only way to stay attached was through a dependent denial of myself and submission to my mother's ways. I don't feel so bad now. I am more Rebecca's mother than the daughter of my mother. . . .
>
> . . . I have become normal. I like myself. I could lose weight after Rebecca was born without fear of anorexia. When I see ballet, I admire the grace of the dancers, but those who are too thin give me a sickly feeling. I have a responsibility to my daughter to avoid bad food habits.
>
> . . . If I were 18 again, I'd want to do it differently. I'd go to college, get all A's and go to medical school and become a pediatrician or child analyst. But I can't do that and I'm not really unhappy.

There was a last looking back at how she became anorectic:

> Something about the whole experience was, and still is, deeply repressed. I was confused. Was the amenorrhea a sign of flowering femininity in the form of a pregnancy or of the opposite—a shutting down? Something was happening physically; it was not up to me; it was out of my hands. One thing is sure—it was a denial of my sexual identity, which wasn't very strong in the first place. That is what is different now as I see myself as Rebecca's mother.

In subsequent years, she and her family moved to a distant state where her husband was happy and successful in his career as well as family life and she at home busy and satisfied caring for their three children.

V

I close with a number of ideas and questions that I had in the course of this psychoanalysis.

Ms. K. was genuinely interested in understanding herself as truly and deeply as she could. She was generally all too ready to find responsibility in herself for what happened in her adult life. After much searching and reflection she continued to describe her experience in anorexia as being caught in a force quite out of her control, like being pulled out to sea in a rip tide. Anorectics can be great rationalizers, and, of course, one cannot be confident that such descriptions by patients reflect more than ignorance or rationalization. Still, I am left with the question of whether such subjective experiences reflect the operation in some restricter anorectics of a biological mechanism for the descent of the set point for body fat such as operates adaptively in the life cycle of animals.

It certainly can be argued that this patient's anorexia was so complicated by, and possibly contributed to, by her transference in analysis that the outcome cannot be viewed as representative or pointing a way that other anorectics can use for mastery or growth. It is very clear that neither pregnancy nor becoming a parent in themselves are curative for anorexia nervosa. Pregnancy is, in fact, often a precipitant of the disease. But, in contrast to most reported anorectics, who wish to and do become mothers despite their anorexia and who then return to more anorectic ways after delivery, this patient used her analysis, her pregnancy, and motherhood as motives and means for overcoming anorexia nervosa.

Most clinicians who know patients with anorexia nervosa are impressed with how completely love relationships and, even, loving feelings are squeezed out of the patients' lives as the disease progresses and the whole emotional life becomes focused on food and body weight. Even in the phase of recovery from weight loss many anorectics are still too preoccupied with these to experience real loving feelings. It is the argument of this paper that the powerful, even if narcissistic, experience of falling in love with a baby and child can provide, in some cases, an opening for the anorectic in therapy to be active in restructuring the sense of self based on a new, positive mother–child relationship that is, probably, in turn based on the parallel experience of finding a positive relationship in the therapy. The patient needs the capacity, often impaired in anorectics, for a strong investment in building and using a positive therapeutic relationship — stronger than the investment in thinness. The therapist needs to be able and willing to foster the growth of such a relationship and help the patient find the opportunity in being a good parent of mastering some of the specific deficits and conflicts that are central in the psychotherapy of anorexia nervosa.

References

Abraham, S., and Beumont, P. (1982), Varieties of psychosexual experience in patients with anorexia nervosa, *Int. J. Eating Disorders, 1,* 10–19.

Bemporad, J., and Ratey, J. (1985), Intensive psychotherapy of former anorexic individuals, *Am. J. Psychotherapy, 39,* 454–466.

Beumont, P., Beardwood, C., and Russell, G. (1972), The occurrence of the syndrome of anorexia nervosa in male subjects, *Psychol. Med., 2,* 216–231.

Beumont, P., Abraham, S., and Simson, K. (1981), The psychosexual histories of adolescent girls and young women with anorexia nervosa, *Psychol. Med., 11,* 131–140.

Bruch, H. (1973), *Eating Disorders,* Basic Books, New York.

Buvat-Herbaut, M., Hebbinckuys, P., Lemaire, A., and Buvat, J. (1983), Attitudes toward weight, body image, menstruation, pregnancy, and sexuality in 81 cases of anorexia compared with 288 normal control school girls, *Int. J. Eating Disorders, 2,* 45–59.

Crisp, A. (1980), *Anorexia Nervosa: Let Me Be,* Grune & Stratton, New York.

Crisp, A., Hsu, L., Chen, C., and Wheeler, M. (1982), Reproductive hormone profiles in male anorexia nervosa before, during and after restoration of body weight to normal, *Int. J. Eating Disorders, 1,* 3–9.

Crisp, A., and Burns, T. (1983), The clinical presentation of anorexia nervosa in the male, *Int. J. Eating Disorders, 2,* 5–10.

Dally, P., and Sargent, W. (1966), Treatment and outcome of anorexia nervosa, *Br. Med. J., 2,* 793–765.

Doolittle, H. (1956), *Tribute to Freud*, Carcanet Press, Oxford, 1971.

Diagnostic and Statistical Manual of Mental Disorders, (3rd Ed. rev) (1987), American Psychiatric Association, Washington, D.C.

Freud, S. (1909), Notes on a case of obsessional neurosis, *Standard Edition*, Hogarth Press, London, 1965. Vol. 10, pp. 153–251.

Garfinkel, P., and Garner, D. (1984), Anorexia nervosa, *Psychiat. Ann.*, *14*, 445.

Kaufman, M., and Heiman, M. (eds.), (1964), *Evolution of Psychosomatic Concepts. Anorexia Nervosa: A Paradigm*, International Universities Press, New York.

Katz, J., Boyar, R., Roffwarg, H., Hellman, L., and Weiner, H. (1978), Weight and circadian luteinizing hormone secretory patterns in anorexia nervosa. *Psychsoma. Med., 40*, 549–567.

Mrosovsky, N., and Sherry, D. (1980), Animal anorexias. *Science, 207*, 837–842.

Namir, S., Melman, K., Yager, J. (1986), Pregnancy in restricter-type anorexia nervosa: a study of six women, *Int. J. Eating Disorders, 5*, 837–845.

Scott, D. (1987), The involvement of psychosexual factors in the causation of eating disorders: Time for a reappraisal, *Int. J. Eating Disorders, 6*, 199–213.

Sours, J. (1980), *Starving to Death in a Sea of Objects*, Jason Aronson, New York.

Stewart, D., and Rankin, J. (1988), Report to American Psychiatric Association Annual Meeting.

Thoma, H. (1967), *Anorexia Nervosa*, Trans. G. Brydone, International Universities Press, New York.

218 Franklin Street
Newton, MA 02158

ANOREXIA NERVOSA IN
THE CONGENITALLY BLIND:
THEORETICAL CONSIDERATIONS

JULES R. BEMPORAD, M.D.
DAVID HOFFMAN, M.D.
DAVID B. HERZOG, M.D.

The recent preoccupation with dieting, exercise, and thinness as a feminine ideal in Western culture has been blamed for the exponential increase in eating disorders in young women. Advertisements, prominent female celebrities, fashion models, and popular publications all tend to present slenderness as equivalent to success and desirability. The number of feature articles on dieting and weight loss in six major women's magazines during the past 20 years has increased, as has the popularity of slender Miss America winners and Playboy centerfolds (Schwartz et al., 1982). The emphasis on appearance, specifically a slim one, is particularly prominent in the teen years. Orbach (1986) notes that "one thing that adolescent magazines uniformly preach as a solution to the crisis of adolescence is dieting and weight control" (p. 47).

The temporal correlation between our cultural fascination with feminine slenderness and the prevalance of eating disorders in women points to a social basis for this form of psychopathology. However, anorexia nervosa existed prior to our modern preoccupation with thinness as an aesthetic ideal. Bruch (1973) found clinical descriptions of anorexia dating back to the 1600s and noted a steady, if modest, stream of reports in the literature since then, including during times when feminine corpulence was highly esteemed. In these cases, it is harder to see how cultural values influenced women to develop eating disorders. These past examples of anorexia may be different from today's cases in terms of etiological conflicts, manifestations, and prognosis. Modern-day anorexia nervosa may represent a final pathway for a variety of developmental difficulties facing contemporary adolescents, difficulties compounded and, perhaps, in some, created by the value

From the Department of Psychiatry, Harvard Medical School (J. R. B.); Massachusetts Mental Health Center (D. Hoffman); and the Massachusetts General Hospital (D. Herzog).

our society places on physical appearance. In contrast, historic instances of anorexia nervosa may consist of a more homogeneous form of illness that was less dependent on social norms or pressures. Those individuals may represent a more pernicious illness with a more severe course than that of a youngster who might go overboard with a fad diet in order to become more attractive or acceptable to others.

It may thus be of interest to explore the occurrence of anorexia nervosa in blind individuals who, presumably, have been less affected by the visual media to achieve or maintain a slender body. Anorexia nervosa has been described, albeit infrequently, in visually impaired individuals. We have found a total of five such cases in the literature. One case involved an adolescent whose visual impairment was secondary to Laurence-Moon-Biedl syndrome (including retinitis pigmentosa, obesity, genital hyperplasia, polydactyly, and mental retardation) and because of these confounding multiple deficits, it will not be described. The other cases are summarized below.

Bruch (1973) reported the case of Olga, who had been "practically blind" since age 10 secondary to uveitis and iritis. She became anorexic at age 12 when her mother, who had been very involved with Olga, decided to pursue interests of her own. Previously, Olga had been on the plump side, possibly due to chronic steriod medication. Despite her visual impairment, Olga was an excellent student, a good athlete, and popular with her peers. According to Bruch, she responded rapidly to family and individual psychotherapy, the latter of which focused on Olga identifying and expressing affect. Bruch comments that the favorable outcome may have been due to the mother's former overinvolvement being based on realistic necessity rather than on a neurotic need to dominate her child, so that Olga was allowed to individuate in a normal manner.

Vandereycken (1986) reported two cases of anorexia in visually handicapped adolescents. Rita was myopic, and had poor vision and nystagmus from birth. She became anorexic at age 16, requiring hospitalization one year later. The author describes Rita as torn between perfectionistic strivings and extreme dependency on her mother. The anorexia developed in the context of Rita's growing awareness of the obstacles she would face in forming heterosexual relationships, which she both desired and feared. Rita was successfully treated with individual psychotherapy, which centered on her attachment–autonomy conflict. Seven years after hospitalization, Rita had no major symptoms of anorexia, although she was still weight conscious. Currently she lives by herself and works as a physiotherapist. Although Rita has an active social life, she remains ambivalent about forming close heterosexual relationships.

Vandereycken's second case is Clare, born blind as a result of an intrauterine rubella infection. She became anorexic shortly after her 14th birthday when, in the course of a routine examination, her doctor commented that she was "a bit too heavy." Clare immediately started dieting, with the same determination and success that typified all of her endeavors. At first Clare was pleased with the positive attention she received from parents and teachers as a result of her weight loss, but she became frightened when she could not stop her dieting voluntarily. She eventually entered a hospital where she improved, particularly after a dramatic family session in which her parents admitted their feelings of guilt regarding their daughter's blindness. Six months after discharge, Clare was reported as doing well in a school for the visually impaired.

Yager et al. (1986) published a case report of a 28-year-old woman who developed anorexia nervosa at age 21, having been blind since age two following surgery and radiation therapy for a neuroblastoma. This woman presented a complex psychiatric history, having been raised by parents who fought constantly and who frequently separated, only to reunite later. The patient recalled that when she began menstruating and physically developing at age 13, she became horrified that she would get fat. She remembered her adolescence as an unhappy time when she felt isolated, depressed, and frequently suicidal. At age 20 she was dismissed from college, where she was studying music, for obscure reasons, possibly relating to her blindness. Feeling increasingly depressed, she was hospitalized and for the first time encountered anorexic women. At first she believed they were "weird," but she also developed the idea of losing weight herself. She began to equate being fat with badness and being thin with goodness, and initiated dieting after leaving the hospital. Since that time the patient has been preoccupied with dieting and weight control. She continues to suffer from numerous depressive episodes that have not responded to a variety of drugs or even a course of electroconvulsive therapy. At the time of her most recent evaluation, this women was found to have a number of personality problems in addition to her anorexic symptoms.

The foregoing summarizes the reported cases of anorexia nervosa in the visually impaired. These individuals raise interesting questions regarding the nature of anorexia nervosa. Vandereycken notes that most studies on body-image development and distortion in eating-disordered individuals have relied on visual perception and have ignored other senses, such as proprioception, which might be more pertinent to blind individuals. He also points out the difficulties that blind individuals might have in developing images of bodies, since touching, presumably the major avenue of such information to them, is socially censured. These difficulties may be particularly acute during adolescence, when bodily changes are most marked. He questions how the blind adolescent can obtain a truthful mirroring of the changes that her body is undergoing. Yager et al. raise related issues, such as the difficulties implicit in early mother–infant interactions without visual communication, and the ramifications of this limitation on the development of the self. The patient they described adopted an anorexic identity only after she became severely depressed and seems to have copied this form of pathological adaptation from others. Dieting and preoccupation with weight control appear to have offered her security and achievement at a time when her vulnerable sense of self was crumbling.

It is of interest that none of the individuals reported seem to have been unduly driven by the cultural idealization of thinness. Therapy focused on issues of individuation and acceptance of the problems that visual impairment presented in adolescence. Little mention is made of body-image distortion or of avoidance of sexuality, although the latter seems to have been a prominent theme in the lives of these women. Similarly, except for the girl described by Bruch, the need to deny or control disturbing affects is not discussed, despite the illness presenting at a time of intense conflict. One probable reason for these omissions is that the cases have been written up in a brief, summarized format without an attempt at a thorough psychodynamic formulation. In view of these intriguing yet unresolved questions, the following case of a women who was congenitally blind and who developed anorexia nervosa in her teens is presented in some detail.

Case History: Lisa

The patient, Lisa, is the third of five children born into a wealthy, midwestern white Catholic family. Her blindness was first noted when she was two weeks old. Lisa's mother had been seriously ill during the first trimester of her pregnancy; although the exact nature of the illness is unknown, it is thought to have resulted in the patient's blindness.

Between the ages of three months and three years, Lisa had a total of ten operations attempting to restore her vision. Despite these interventions, her vision remains limited to faint light perception in one eye. The patient relates a number of prominent memories to this series of traumatic events. She vividly recalls the smell of the anesthetic ether, describing it as the "most nauseous substance in the world." Ether would make her "blow up like a balloon," and upon regaining consciousness after each operation, she would vomit. To this day she has nightmares about these early experiences in which an unidentified person of unknown gender tries to smother her with an ether-scented mattress. She states that ether smells like "death," but is unable to elaborate further as to what this means to her, except that it terrifies her.

Lisa has few fond memories of her mother, with whom she has had minimal contact during her adult life. The patient remembers her mother telling her she was the worst baby that she had nursed. Mother is described as being cold and distant, a "visually oriented perfectionist" who is "exceedingly dependent on her husband." The patient feels that her mother was completely intolerant of her blindness. Mother would comment sarcastically on the ugliness of Lisa's clothing (i.e., not being color coordinated) and point out the "disgusting" and inappropriate facial expressions of the patient. In order to avoid her mother's ridicule, Lisa learned to control her body and facial movements to such an uncanny degree that, today, a casual observer would not notice that she was blind. Many clinicians have expressed the suspicion that she must be malingering. In fact, Lisa is able to toss a ball into a wastebasket across a room if the latter is tapped only once to reveal its location. Lisa's quest to satisfy her mother's demands that she not behave like a blind person had driven her to acquire a vast knowledge of the visual arts. She also dresses in impeccably color coordinated outfits. One of the few relatives she remembers with fondness is her maternal aunt, who taught her about colors.

Father is described as a successful businessman who is "domineering" and "jealous." Lisa claims that he promoted dependency in his wife and other children by supporting them financially. However, she also remembers him as the more nurturing and supportive parent during her childhood. A significant early memory involves being accidentally hit in the head by a baseball bat and feeling terrified that her eyes had been knocked out. She ran crying to her mother for comfort, but it was her father who eventually picked her up and held her. Later childhood memories of her father reveal an uneasiness over his attempts at physical closeness. When Lisa was 11 or 12 and visited her family on occasional weekends, her father would pinch her waist. She found his touching her as "intrusive" and "obscene," thinking to herself that he should not be doing such things to her. However, she never verbalized her displeasure.

Of her siblings, Lisa was close only to one older sister, Joan, who functioned as a kind of surrogate mother during her first five years, caring for her, holding her, and, at times, even letting her sleep in her bed. When Lisa felt scared or insecure, or had just awoken from a nightmare, it was to Joan that she went to for comfort. Lisa would turn to Joan for relief from a pervasive fear that she developed in early childhood. This fear focused on her contracting poliomyelitis, becoming paralyzed, and having to live out her days in an iron lung. The thought of her losing control of her body was understandably horrifying. The origin of this fear is uncertain, except that there was concern in the family about the children possibly acquiring polio from swimming pools. Her aunt commented that Joan was like a "little mother" to Lisa and, indeed, Joan is the only one in the family remembered as nurturing. Lisa's younger brothers seem to have not played a significant role in her development.

Another sister later developed bulimia, indicating some familial predisposition toward eating disorders. There was, in the mother's system of values, a correlation between obesity and either unhappiness or mental illness. Obese individuals somehow were unable to cope successfully with life. While the mother was not overly thin, she struggled not to become fat, being a member of Weight Watchers and carefully keeping to a diet.

The patient achieved her early developmental milestones normally. In fact, at age five when she was sent to a state boarding school for blind children, she was more intellectually and physically adept than most of her peers. She excelled academically and formed several satisfying friendships with girls her own age. However, she continued to experience nightmares about ether that would awaken the other children, and consequently had to be separated from the other girls and slept in a separate room. She developed an intense fear of vomiting in reaction to another student who exhibited projectile vomiting shortly before dying of a brain tumor. Between the ages of eight and ten, Lisa had recurring stomach aches that she feared would result in vomiting. To cope with the stomach aches, she developed a compulsive ritual that involved spelling words on her fingers. A school psychologist helped her with both her stomach aches and the compulsive behavior. Lisa does not remember any sexual feelings during her years at the boarding school, and denies having had crushes on any of her school mates. However, she alluded repeatedly to an episode of sexual abuse at age six while she was at boarding school, but declined to elaborate.

Aside from the instances of fear described above and the recurrence of terrifying nightmares, Lisa admits to experiencing little or no feeling. She describes herself as "alexithymic," being unable to identify or feel emotions since early childhood. Similarly, she states that she has never experienced any sexual desires nor elaborated sexual fantasies.

The main nurturing figures at the boarding school were the house mothers. Lisa remembers feeling that many of them seemed put out by how difficult she could be, and that it was wrong to ask them for help because the other children had more trouble dressing themselves than she did. However, she felt that several of the house mothers were caring people who genuinely liked her. During this time at boarding school, the patient felt acutely rejected by her parents. Whereas most of the children spent every weekend at home, she spent only every other weekend with her family, at most. She became increasingly estranged from her nurturant sister, and experienced repeated examples of what she felt was rejecting behavior by her parents such as when her father, in a rush to return home from the airport near school, "flagged down the first car that drove by," and had the driver take her back to the school. While her classmates received mail almost every day, Lisa's mother wrote her only once a week. She interpreted her parent's actions by assuming she had done something wrong and deserved to be given less.

Because she was such an exceptional pupil, Lisa was selected to be a trial student in a "mainstreaming" program, and at age 15 moved back home and began attending public school. It was at this point that she first started to manifest serious psychiatric difficulties. This transition proved extremely disturbing for a number of reasons. Her family did little to welcome her at home and seemed to resent her presence. For example, her mother refused to take Lisa shopping because, according to Lisa, she was embarrassed to be seen with her. Her sister, who was in the same high school, also seemed embarrassed at having a blind relative. At school she felt confused and lost among sighted peers. She did not understand jokes or idioms that relied on the sense of vision. Lisa believed that other students avoided her and found her repulsive. If some acted kindly, she interpreted this behavior as condescending or pitying toward her. She did well academically but otherwise shunned contact with any school activities. She withdrew more and more, feeling panicky, depressed, and confused. Her home offered little refuge or respite. In that setting she felt she could do nothing correctly. She feared wearing clothes that did not match and so incur her mother's criticism. In addition, her mother was a fanatic housekeeper and Lisa was frightened that she might leave her possessions around the house or get things dirty without knowing it.

Apparently her parents ignored her progressive deterioration, but her aunt who visited often was disturbed by Lisa's depression and withdrawal. This aunt confronted Lisa's father, while Lisa eavesdropped, asking him to "do something" to help his daughter. The father angrily replied that Lisa's problems were her own "damn fault" and that Lisa had to "pull herself up by her own bootstraps."

Her father's comments completely shattered Lisa's sense of self. To this day, she recalls them as if they were just uttered. She could not face the fact that her father cared so little about her or that she was such a weakling in his eyes. She wanted to die and, indeed, attempted suicide by ingesting a number of pills. This desperate act forced her parents to bring Lisa for psychiatric help. She recalls really liking her therapist but being unable to talk to him. She did not want him to see her because she felt ugly and repulsive, both in terms of her appearance and as a human being. She was convinced she was weak, completely unlikable, and possibly evil. At the time, she only wanted to die.

This was the context in which Lisa developed anorexia nervosa. She did so without knowing that such an illness existed or ever hearing about thinness being equated with greater acceptance or desirability. She states that she was not affected consciously by her mother equating corpulence with unhappiness. Lisa describes her anorexic behavior as "just happening." She continued in therapy for the next three years, with worsening anorexia and frequent suicide attempts.

At age 18, Lisa recalls meeting someone who, for the first time, accepted her blindness and her emaciated state. Lisa had a close emotional and romantic affair with this woman, adopting many of her attitudes and values. Unfortunately, this woman was killed in an automobile accident less than one year after the relationship began. Following her loss, Lisa had to be hospitalized in a quasi-psychotic state. During this inpatient stay, nasogastric tube feeding had to be used to stem Lisa's progressive cachexia. Such feedings were exceedingly terrifying for Lisa who sensed she had lost all control of her body and imagined she would swell up like a balloon. She taught herself to vomit, despite her fear of this act, in order to stop her tube feedings. In this manner, Lisa was able to eat, demonstrating that she no longer required tube feedings, and then vomit in secret. Since this hospitalization, Lisa has persisted in vomiting many times each day. She describes the experience as "horrible" yet uncontrollable. The induced emesis has allowed her to eat somewhat adequately yet maintain a subnormal weight for her stature.

The only other notable relationship in Lisa's history was with a charismatic older man who led an organization for the advancement and care of the blind. Lisa met him shortly after discharge from the above hospitalization and responded to his pressure and expectation that she achieve more for herself and for all blind individuals. Under his tutelage, Lisa worked hard lecturing and lobbying for the organization and later attended college. She describes this man as gruff, demanding, but very attentive. The time Lisa spent working with him probably represents her period of optimal functioning. Under the close scrutiny of a strict but charismatic male mentor, she was free of disabling psychiatric symptoms for two years. However, when she separated from him to attend college at his urging, Lisa could not function and had to withdraw from school.

Since that time, Lisa has done poorly. Her anorexia has continued unabated. There have been numerous hospitalizations, primarily for suicide attempts. She states that she hates herself for disappointing others, for being "an elephantine blob," and for having little purpose or accomplishments in her life. At present, Lisa denies any active fantasy life or dreams. She says she feels empty inside. She is obsessed with her weight and claims to know exactly how much she weighs each day just by how her body feels. Her relationships are marked by a profound ambivalence and ultimately are self-limited. In general, she tries to present a complaint yet self-reliant facade, while in her therapeutic relationships she has become exceedingly dependent and desirous of nurturance, traits that she considers disgusting and immoral. She is a meticulous housekeeper, dresses fashionably, can be quite witty, and, at times, even charming, yet is chronically depressed and is constantly on the verge of self-destruction.

DISCUSSION

Despite being congenitally blind, Lisa's history and course are quite similar to those of numerous sighted anorexics. As one traces her development, experiences are encountered that have been identified in the literature as characteristic of the premorbid life of women who succumb to this disorder. Lisa's family constellation, including a mother who has difficulty giving to others in a genuine way, while maintaining a facade of self-sacrifice; and a father who needs to control others and to exact from others a reflected self-image of powerful masculinity, has been noted by Gordon et al. (this issue), as well as Bemporad and Ratey (1985). In listening to Lisa recount her past, the interviewer senses that behind the numerous historical events, a core theme that recurs is the lack of parental appreciation for Lisa as a whole person and her acceptance only in the guise of a socially acceptable facade that reflected predominantly the needs of the parents. This lack of empathic acknowledgment in the causation of anorexia nervosa has been described by Bruch (1973) in her seminal contributions and more recently documented convincingly by Geist (1984) in his examination of this disorder in the framework of Kohut's self psychology.

Other pertinent historical events that may have influenced Lisa's pathology but are not uniformly found in the past of sighted anorexics include her series of operations in early life. These must have been experienced as highly traumatic, as they appear responsible for her childhood fear of body paralysis (secondary to poliomyelitis), and her recurrent nightmares about ether that continue to this day. These early experiences of bodily assault and loss of control certainly would suggest the creation of defensive overvigilance and overcontrol regarding bodily functions. However, it is also apparent from the psychological residua of the repeated surgery that not much was offered by the parents to ease Lisa'a understandable panic and terror.

Lisa's role in the family is also not typical of most future anorexics. Minuchin et al. (1978), for example, portray the anorexic as playing a pivotal role in her family's disturbed equilibrium. These authors suggest that the psychosomatogenic family needs the symptom-bearing child in order to avoid confronting or resolving conflicts and to pretend that their difficulties emanate from the child's physical illness. In contrast, Lisa seems to have been an embarrassment to her family who wished her not to exist at all. It may be that her lack of role in the family, be it pathological or healthy, accounts for Lisa's considerable personality pathology, in addition to her problems related to anorexia. An alternative possibility may be that in some families of anorexics, even a part of those described by Minuchin, there is a destructive wish toward the child beneath the more apparent exploitative use of the child's illness.

What is known is that even before starting boarding school at age five, Lisa was already socially and intellectually precocious, a characteristic described by Geist (1984) as exhibiting the future anorexic's conditional acceptance and early development of an extensive false self. This facade, developed to please powerful others as well as to repress dependency needs, seems to have continued and even flourished in boarding school. By the time Lisa returned home in early adolescence, she had consolidated a character structure typical of severe anorexics: lack of feeling, need for control, perfectionism, distrust of others, and a pervasive anhedonia. Her return to a world of sighted individuals challenged and, ultimately, defeated her already pathological mode of coping. Her need for status and emotionless, efficient functioning could no longer be maintained. She was assaulted by demands that were beyond her capabilities, much as is seen in situations that characterize the onset of anorexia in sighted individuals. Similarly, the family was of little emotional support in these most trying times. Lisa repeatedly recited the critical words of her father and her resultant profound disappointment in his reaction to her helplessness, almost in the manner of someone with post-traumatic stress disorder. The memory of his belittling of her efforts is still vivid and painful to her. Guidano and Liotti (1983) and Bemporad and Ratey (1985) have noted a disillusionment with the father as a not infrequent event in the onset of this disorder. It is as if this rejection of oneself is the last straw in a series of painful rebuffs and self-perceived failures to function adequately.

Following this devastating rebuff, Lisa experienced almost total despair and her fragile and specious sense of self was further shattered when her family refused to respond to her even more desperate state. In this context, Lisa somehow hit upon anorexia as a means of regaining a sense of control over her inner life. If her memory is accurate, Lisa had no knowledge of this disorder nor did she consider slenderness as desirable (despite her mother's weight consciousness). Neither does there seem to have been any initial positive reinforcement from others for weight reduction. Her self-starvation appears to have developed as the last-ditch attempt to gain some sort of mastery and to distract herself from her profound dysphoria and anxiety. It seems to have been the final attempt to preserve her facade/false self of detached, perfectionistic, and counterdependent strivings. Once launched, Lisa's anorexia took on a life of its own, continuing to be used to perpetuate her pathological mode of being.

So much of Lisa's history is congruent with that of other individuals with severe, persistant anorexia nervosa, that it seems difficult to find a role for her blindness in the etiology of her illness. Blindness would seem to make the child more dependent on caretakers and, in Lisa's case, cause a more desperate defensive counterdependent stance. However, in most cases of uncomplicated congenital blindness, the parents compensate for their child's deficit so that according to Blank (1957), Cooper (1979), Burlingham (1972), and Fraiberg and Freeman (1964), most blind children grow up as psychologically healthy. The theoretical importance of Lisa's blindness as regards the pathogenesis of anorexia nervosa is that it prevented her from being influenced by the social idealization of thinness and the positing of thinness as a way of solving psychological problems. For Lisa, the creation of anorexia was more an escape from inner turmoil and a defenseive maneuver against feelings of failure and internal fragmentation than the deliberate expression of a wish to become more popular, beautiful, or desirable. Her particular case indicates that some forms of eating disorders, perhaps those with a poorer prognosis, are independent of cultural conceptions of feminine appearance. Lisa, as with some of her sighted counterparts, with whom she shares similar conflicts and developmental pathology, strongly suggests that true anorexia nervosa, in any historical context, is a disorder of impaired object relations and of a defective conceptualization of the self.

References

Bemporad, J. R., and Ratey, J. (1985), Intensive psychotherapy of former anorexic individuals, *Am. J. Psychother., 39*, 454–465.

Blank, H. R. (1957), Psychoanalysis and blindness, *Psychoanal. Quart., 26*, 1–24.

Bruch, H. (1983), *Eating Disorders*, Basic Books, New York.

Burlingham, D. (1972), *Psychoanalytic Studies of the Sighted and the Blind*, International Universities Press, New York.

Cooper, A. F., (1979), The psychological problems of the deaf and blind, *Scottish Med. J., 24*, 105–107.

Dunn, T. L., and Coorey, P. R. (1982), Anorexia nervosa, visual disturbance and Lawrence-Moon-Biedl syndrome (letter), *Lancet, 1*, 1184.

Fraiberg, S., and Freedman, D. A. (1964), Studies in the ego development of the congenitally blind child, *Psychoanal. Study Child, 19*, 113–169.

Geist, R. A. (1984), Psychotherapeutic dilemmas in the treatment of anorexia nervosa: A self-psychological perspective, *Contemp. Psychother. Rev., 2*, 268–288.

Gordon, C., Beresin, E., Herzog, D. (1989), The parents' relationship and the child's illness in anorexia nervosa, *J. Amer. Acad. Psychoanal., 17*, 29–42.

Guidano, V. F., and Liotti, G. (1983), *Cognitive Processes and Emotional Disorders*, Guilford Press, New York.

Minuchin, S., Rosman, B. L., and Baker, L. (1978), *Psychosomatic Families*, Harvard University Press, Cambridge.

Orbach, S. (1986), *Hunger Strike*, W. W. Norton, New York.

Schwartz, D. M., Thompson, M. G., and Johnson, C. L. (1982), Anorexia and bulimia: The socio-cultural context. *Int. J. Eating Disorders, 1*, 20–36.

Vandereycken, W. (1986), Anorexia nervosa and visual impairment. *Comp. Psychiatry, 27*, 545–548.

Yager, J., Hatton, C. A., and Ma, L. (1986), Anorexia nervosa in a woman totally blind since the age of two, *Brit. J. Psychiatry, 149*, 506–509.

74 Fenwood Road
Boston, MA 02115

THE PROCESS OF RECOVERING
FROM ANOREXIA NERVOSA

EUGENE V. BERESIN, M.D.
CHRISTOPHER GORDON, M.D.
DAVID B. HERZOG, M.D.

The authors describe the process of recovering from anorexia nervosa as it is revealed by 13 women who have recovered from the illness. Emphasizing the patient's perspective, the paper reviews the perceived causes of the disorder,
helpful and harmful therapy-related and life experiences,
features hardest to change, the defensive function of anorexia nervosa and residual traits. Generally, the movement
toward health entails forming a therapeutic relationship in
which the anorexic can identify and express feelings, experience the empathic, nonjudgmental understanding of another person, separate from a pathological family system,
resolve hostile dependent attachment to parents, assuage
primitive guilt, and engage in the trials of adolescent psychosexual development to enter adulthood with the beginnings of a firm, cohesive sense of self.

"What is REAL?" asked the Rabbit one day, when they were lying side
by side near the nursery fender, before Nana came to tidy the room. "Does
it mean having things that buzz inside you and a stick-out handle?"

"Real isn't how you are made," said the Skin Horse. "It's a thing that
happens to you when a child loves you for a long, long time, not just to play
with but REALLY loves you, then you become Real."

"Does it hurt?" asked the Rabbit.

"Sometimes," said the Skin Horse, for he was always truthful. "When
you are Real you don't mind being hurt."

Eugene V. Beresin and David Herzog are with the Child Psychiatry Service,
Massachusetts General Hospital; and Christopher Gordon is with the Human
Resource Institute, Brookline.

The authors wish to thank the subjects of this study and acknowledge their
honesty, compassion, and determination to assist clinicians and patients struggling with anorexia nervosa. We also appreciate Debby Redifer's help in preparing
the manuscript and Julie Eisenstein's valuable interpretation of statistical tests.

"Does it happen all at once, like being wound up," he asked, "or bit by bit?"

"It doesn't happen all at once," said the Skin Horse. "You become. It takes a long time. That's why it doesn't often happen to people who break easily, or have sharp edges or who have to be carefully kept. Generally, by the time you are Real, most of your hair has been loved off, and your eyes drop out and you get loose in the joints and very shabby. But these things don't matter at all, because once you are Real you can't be ugly, except to people who don't understand." — Margery Williams, *The Velveteen Rabbit*

Clinicians who work with anorexic patients over the long term may be fortunate to witness a remarkable transformation not unlike the Velveteen Rabbit's. Throughout the illness, these sensitive young women deny and defy life in their abrogation of feelings, reversal of normal psychobiologic development, monk-like asceticism, rigid, mechanistic rituals, empty black-and-white formulas for appearance and behavior, and social isolation. Anorexia nervosa is a defensive retreat from the world of the living, which is viewed and experienced as exploitative, unempathic, dangerous, and untrustworthy. Like the Velveteen Rabbit, they do not feel real or understand the process of becoming a real, feeling person, but imagine it to be a mechanical activity and fear being hurt. They are the ones, aptly described by the Skin Horse, who break easily, have sharp edges, and are carefully kept in their families. They do not experience being truly loved for themselves, and instead of withstanding the expectable bruises and failures in healthy intimate relationships, feel they must be beautiful, perfect, and compliant to be loved. Indeed, they feel ugly — intolerant of their inner hurt, envy, rage, and primitive guilt, ensconced in a world of people who do not understand. Most clinicians would concur that becoming real is a gradual, bit-by-bit metamorphosis, taking a long time. But how does this becoming happen? Let us first try to answer this by looking at the research literature.

Despite the common intractability of anorexia nervosa, some patients do recover to lead relatively normal lives. Outcome studies (Bruch, 1973; Crisp, 1983a; Garfinkel and Garner, 1982; Hall et al., 1984; Hsu, 1980; Morgan and Russell, 1975; Morgan et al., 1983; Rollins and Piazza, 1981; Schwartz and Thompson, 1981) are summarized in Table 1. It is evident from the data that considering weight, menses, eating attitudes and behavior, psychosexual functioning, interpersonal and family relationships, work history, and psychiatric symptoms, only 40% are totally recovered and

Table 1.   Summary of Outcome Studies

Weight: >50% maintain weight within 15% of average
Menses: >50% menstruate (all have normal weight; some with normal weight
  fail to menstruate)
Eating Attitudes: 35% have "normal" eating attitudes
Eating Behavior: 35% have "normal" eating behavior
Psychosexual Function: 60% have "normal" sexual attitudes and behavior
  50% eventually marry or live with significant other
Interpersonal Relationships (outside family):
  60% maintain satisfying social relations
  25–45% express social anxiety (usually increases as weight increases)
Family Relationships: 40–55% have persistent family problems. Most commonly:
  emotional dependency with hostility and resentment toward family even
  after weight recovery
Work History: >70% have good work histories even at low weight
Psychiatric Symptoms: 20–40% complain of depression
  5–20% complain of obsessions
  10–40% complain of social phobia
  More frequent in non-weight-recovered subjects or if weight recovered,
  subjects with abnormal eating attitudes and behavior.
Global Outcome (Garfinkel and Garner, 1982): 40% totally recovered
  30% improved
  30% die or are chronically
  affected

References: Bruch, 1973; Crisp, 1983a; Garfinkel and Garner, 1982; Hall et al., 1984; Hsu, 1980; Morgan and Russell, 1975; Rollins and Piazza, 1981; Schwartz and Thompson, 1981.

another 30% are improved with some disability in the above-noted variables (Garfinkel and Garner, 1982). However, reviews of outcome studies by Garfinkel and Garner (1982), Hsu (1980) and Schwartz and Thompson (1981) indicate significant discrepancies in the results of different studies, and it is not clear whether these are due to problems in research methods or to clinical features that have not been effectively studied (e.g., individual biological, psychological, or social/environmental differences, comparison of treatment techniques, impact of life events). Moreover, there is considerable disagreement among researchers on prognostic indicators (Garfinkel and Garner, 1982).

Some of these research problems arise from inadequate definitions of the illness and recovery. The DSM-III-R diagnostic criteria for anorexia nervosa do not include some of the most disabling features of the disorder, for example, social impairment, low self-esteem, disturbed family relations, delayed psychosexual development, and psychiatric symptoms including depression, anxiety, social phobias, obsessions, and compulsions. Most outcome studies have not explored the rich psychodynamic literature regarding family psychopathology (Bemporad and Ratey, 1985; Crisp, 1983b; Minuchin et al., 1978; Palazzoli, 1978), impaired object relations (Masterson, 1977; Palazzoli, 1978; Piazza et al., 1980; Rollins and Blackwell, 1968; Sours, 1980; Sugarman and Kurash, 1982), character disorders (Johnson and Connors, 1987; Masterson, 1977), or deficits in the self (Bruch, 1982; Geist, 1985; Goodsitt, 1983, 1985; Rizzuto, 1985; Rizzuto et al., 1981; Swift and Letven, 1984). Compounding the problems of defining the illness are difficulties in assessing recovery. Studies have demonstrated that "normal" adolescents eat in an irregular manner (Crisp, 1983a). A large percentage of the adolescent and adult population is excessively concerned with diet, appearance, and weight. Normality is difficult to define, not just in eating attitudes and behavior, but in psychosocial functioning in general.

The research literature is also severely limited in discerning the effect of treatment on outcome. Crisp (1983a), Garfinkel and Garner (1982), and Morgan and Russell (1975) conclude that it is not known whether treatment alters the long-term course of the illness. Since multiple treatments with differing philosophies, orientations, and methods have all produced similar results, some investigators wonder if treatment is unrelated to recovery (Bassoe and Eskeland, 1982; Dally, 1969; Niskanen et al., 1974; Nussbaum et al., 1985; Yager et al., 1987), and whether there is a natural history of the illness, with "spontaneous recovery" (Bassoe and Eskeland, 1982) independent of treatment.

As we reviewed the literature on outcome of anorexia nervosa, we were struck by another deficit. In the effort to obtain quantifiable, replicable outcome measures, somehow the phenomenology of the subject's experience was lost. Nowhere did the studies convey the anorexic's experience of change and recovery. We began reexamining the question of recovery by relying on a basic clinical principal: First and foremost, listen to and understand the patient from her perspective. When viewed in this way, the literature neglects some critical questions regarding the process of recovery:

1. Do you have any idea what caused your anorexia nervosa?
2. How were you able to recover from anorexia nervosa? What

experiences were most helpful and harmful in recovering (both treatment and non-treatment related)?
3. What features of the eating disorder are hardest to change?
4. What did you lose by giving up your anorexia nervosa? What took its place?
5. Do people ever fully recover from anorexia nervosa? What is left?
6. What advice would you give to others who are suffering from anorexia nervosa?

We embarked on a pilot investigation by approaching people who had successfully traversed the battlefield of anorexia nervosa, asking them directly about their experiences.

A PILOT STUDY OF THE PROCESS OF RECOVERING

Method

We placed ads in a local newsletter of an organization devoted to helping eating-disordered patients and their families. Our expressed interest was to study women who once had anorexia nervosa and who now consider themselves recovered to learn more about the process of getting well. We included 13 subjects in the project who previously met DSM-III criteria for anorexia nervosa and now had recovered, based on our examination of the following clinical instruments:
1. Comprehensive Eating Disorders Questionnaire (Massachusetts General Hospital, Eating Disorders Unit)
2. Eating Disorders Inventory (EDI) (Garner et al., 1983)
3. Social Adjustment Scale—Self Report (SAS-SR) (Weissman and Bothwell, 1976; Weissman et al., 1978)
4. Semistructured Clinical Interview (Beresin, Gordon, Herzog)

In the 90-minute semistructured interview, we asked the six questions noted above, reviewed the course of the illness, and discussed answers to the Comprehensive Eating Disorders Questionnaire (which included a detailed personal and family psychosocial history, assessment of current condition, medical and psychiatric history, and eating disorder history). We asked specifically about which features of a wide variety of treatments were helpful or harmful regarding the eating disorder and what non-therapy-related experiences were helpful or harmful. Subjects were asked to rate treatment experiences, including individual psychotherapy, family therapy, group therapy, self-help groups, medications, and hospitalization. Finally, subjects were asked to rank order the five most helpful and harmful treatment-related and non-treatment-related experiences in the process of recovering. After the interview, we rated the subjects globally on the basis of five subscales: eating behaviors, eating attitudes, social involvement, sexual activity/maturity, and separation from family. Each subscale was scored as follows: 1=normal range, 2=minimal impairment, 3=moderate impairment, 4=severe impairment. We established global ratings by averaging the 5 subscale scores. Global ratings were calculated both for the subject's worst condition during the course of her eating disorder based on her history and for her current status.

Our subjects were all Caucasian women with a mean age of 29.4 years. Seven were single, three were divorced, and three were married. The mean age of onset of anorexia nervosa was 16.8 years. Table 2 summarizes the group's course of anorexia nervosa. At one point these women were all severely ill with anorexia nervosa. The average weight loss was 40% below average weight for height and age. All fasted, became amenorrheic, and virtually all had binge episodes with about half purging. Two-thirds abused laxatives and

Table 2.   Pilot Study: Course of Anorexia Nervosa ($n = 13$)

Variable	Past (Means)	Current (Means)
Age of onset	16.8 years	
Weight	60.8%	90.7% (% of average weight for age and height)
Fasting	100%	7.7% (1 subject, rarely)
Bulimia	92.3%	0%
Vomiting	46.2%	7.7% (1 subject, rarely)
Laxatives	76.9%	7.7% (1 subject, rarely)
Diuretics	38.5%	0%
Shoplift Food	30.8%	0%
Amenorrhea	100% (at low weight)	15.4% (1 subject had hysterectomy, 1 subject normal weight without menses)
Global Clinical Rating:*	4.0 (at worst)	1.7 (current)

*Global Clinical Rating: Rating by interviewers including 5 subscales: eating behavior, eating attitudes, social involvement, sexual activity/maturity, separation from family. Each subscale rated from 1=normal range, 2=minimal impairment to 4=severe impairment. Global rating is the average of 5 subscale scores.

approximately one-third abused diuretics. The group's psychiatric history further corroborates the severity of psychopathology. Close to two-thirds of the subjects had a previous psychiatric history other than anorexia nervosa, with over one-third suffering from depression and attempting suicide. Three subjects were hospitalized for disturbances other than eating disorders. Most investigators would agree that this cohort represents a severely impaired, poor prognostic group.

A study of this kind has many limitations. We are only examining a small group with a possible sampling bias, in that the subjects responded to a request for participation. However, all the subjects clearly had a severe illness with clinical features typical of subjects in most outcome studies. There is also potential interviewer bias, since we did not use a standardized interviewing instrument. Interviewer bias is diminished by our long history of working together, familiarity with each other's clinical technique and independent review of each subject's test and interview reports. Finally, we are not able to draw causal or predictive conclusions, since the material is all self-reported.

Apart from these drawbacks and disclaimers, we see clear benefits from the study. The findings may lead to new directions for future outcome research. Above all, the study permits a real appreciation of the patient's perspective. Bruch (1973) notes, in agreement with Palazzoli, that outcome "is entirely dependent on the therapist's capacity to understand the basic problems of the anorexic and to help him find better ways of dealing with them" (p. 381). We hope this investigation will enhance this needed understanding.

Clinical Findings

The 13 subjects had indeed recovered from anorexia nervosa. As a group, the mean weight was about 91% of average weight for age and height, all but two had regular menses (and one of these had a hysterectomy), no one binged, one subject fasted rarely, and one subject vomited on rare occasions. All subjects were employed at an appropriate level. Although we rated the group severely impaired (4.0) globally at its worst, we placed the group in the normal to minimally impaired range (1.7) at the time of the study. The SAS-SR and EDI profiles corroborated this level of recovery, and will be described in some detail below. Overall, we were impressed by the subjects' willingness to reveal themselves and their life histories, honesty and clarity in presenting the course of their illnesses, depth of personal insight, ability to enjoy themselves and their relationships, and compassion for others suffering from anorexia nervosa.

Standard Instruments

The Social Adjustment Scale consists of seven subscales: Work, Social and Leisure, Extended Family, Marital-As Spouse, Parental, Family Unit, and Economic. Each subscale is rated and a global rating is derived from the average of all subscale scores. Compared with normal female controls, our subjects' scores were not significantly different on the global ratings and on all subscale scores except Extended Family ($p < .001$). The Extended Family subscale includes questions about parents, siblings, in-laws, and children not living at home. When we compared our subjects' responses to individual items on the Extended Family scale with those of normal female controls, we noted significant differences in feelings of Rebellion ($p < .01$), Guilt ($p < .01$) and Resentment ($p < .05$). On other individual questions from all other subscales, responses were not significantly different from normal female controls' except for three items on the Social and Leisure subscale: Diminished Social Interactions ($p < .02$), Friction ($p < .01$) and Social Discomfort ($p < .01$). These results are consistent with previous indications that among recovered patients there remains persistent social anxiety (Hsu et al., 1979) and unresolved hostile dependent feelings in the family (Hsu et al., 1979; Morgan and Russell, 1975).

The Eating Disorders Inventory has eight subscales: Drive for Thinness, Bulimia, Body Dissatisfaction, Ineffectiveness, Perfectionism, Interpersonal Distrust, Interoceptive Awareness, and Maturity Fears. No global rating is calculated. We compared our subjects with two control groups provided by the Inventory, female college students and recovered anorexics. We noted no significant differences between our subjects and both control groups on any subscale, except Perfectionism. Here there were significant differences with each: subject vs. female college students ($p < .01$), subject vs. recovered anorexics ($p < .05$). In an attempt to understand this difference, we looked at the individual questions. Of all 64 questions on the EDI the only ones related specifically to family are those on the Perfectionism subscale, and three of the six items are family-related questions: "Only outstanding performance is good enough in my family," "As a child, I tried very hard to avoid disappointing my parents and teachers," and "My parents have expected excellence of me."

We offer three possible interpretations of the differences in Perfectionism. First, subjects who volunteered for this study could be skewed in the direction of greater perfectionism, with participation validating the high achievement of recovery. Other reasons for differences may relate to family issues. The Perfectionism subscale might measure current unresolved family pressures and conflicts, in concert with the SAS findings; or, this scale may indicate increased awareness or understanding of family dynamics that may be a part of the group's recovery.

Perceived Causes of Anorexia Nervosa

All of the subjects attributed the anorexia nervosa to deeply ingrained family conflicts and the roles they played in the family. Although they came from homes with more than ample material means and opportunities for growth and advancement, they found themselves trapped in an enmeshed, overly protective, rigid family system, characterized by covert marital conflict that demanded their active involvement as symptom bearer, confidant, or peacemaker. They felt that they were the glue holding the family together. Their paradigm of relationships, exemplified by their parents, is one of mutual distrust, lacking intimacy and bound by hostile dependency and reaction formation. On the surface everything looked fine, but somehow they knew that appearances were deceiving.

Their mothers were seen as superficially angelic, self-sacrificing, and endlessly giving, yet this demeanor cloaked a fragile, critical, narcissistically vulnerable woman who repudiated her rage through reactive generosity (Gordon et al., this issue; Kernberg, 1980). These mothers could not tolerate the child's growing need to test her aggression during separation and instead demanded peaceful compliance. Most mothers were terribly intrusive, overinvolved, excessively concerned with appearances, and unable to empathically mirror the child's growing needs and abilities. Instead, they imposed their own needs. As young girls, the subjects realized they could not get the nurturance and validation they needed from mother and were profoundly envious and angry. Yet, because of mother's fragility, they could neither own nor express their rage, and, as their mother, lived through reaction formation and false complicity, projecting the rage for fear of hurting someone. As one subject described:

> Mother cloned me. I did what she wanted, when she wanted it and it made her so happy and it made me happy. "Oh, isn't she wonderful," said my mother all the time. I'm a victim, but I also got stroked unconditionally. As a teenager my mother told me what to want, what to wear, to wear this bra or that bra. She was very, very intrusive. I felt I couldn't control anything in my life. I confused nurturance and food. I couldn't get angry, because it would be like destroying someone else, like Mother. It felt like she would hate me forever. I got angry through anorexia nervosa. It was my last hope. It's my own body and this was my last ditch effort.

In another subject's words:

> . . . her idea of selflessness was martyrdom. She was overprotective and gave too much. She very much wanted her family to look good primarily for her own mother and for society in general. She was extremely concerned about what people thought about her, her family, and what people would say about them. She tried to create the perfect family by giving material things but did not develop our soul, spirit, insides, respecting or exploring our opinions. She couldn't do it because she didn't know it herself.

The fathers were typically seen as strong, distant, and successful men, often overinvolved with work to the exclusion of family. Most of these men were at times volatile and prone to use alcohol heavily. The daughters developed strong Oedipal ties to them, usually precociously, to attend to their fathers' narcissism and in the hope of getting the nurturance they lacked from their mothers. The role of "Daddy's little girl," however, was fraught with danger because of the risk of injuring their vulnerable mothers through competition. The fathers were later viewed as terribly needy men who tended to dominate and control their wives out of counterdependency. In short, life at home was terrifying. Underlying the mother's generosity and involvement was voracious greed and rage; beneath the father's powerful facade was low self-esteem, dependency, and misogyny. Feelings were disavowed, particularly aggression, and in the guise of a happy, peaceful household there was tremendous pervasive tension.

The tenacity with which these girls tied themselves to their families was partially due to loyalty and the covert demands parents placed on them, and because of profound deficits in the cohesiveness of their selves. They were unable to tolerate ambivalence in relationships, the lability of feelings, or the struggles with identity and self-concept required in the ascendancy of adolescence:

> I really didn't want to grow up and be independent. I really had no idea how to take care of myself. In that way, I kept myself very dependent and a center of attention. I came from a family where my mother was very dependent on my father. My father was very restrictive. He wanted me to be dependent on him and he enjoyed that. He never encouraged me to do things on my own. I had very few friends and no social network. I was completely alone.

Nor were they prepared for the development of adult sexuality. Many feared recapitulating their parents' relationship:

> . . . anorexia developed because of the type of person I am, energetic, sensitive, obsessive and these features can feed into the disorder. Secondly, I denied my feelings and the role I played in my family. This was especially important. I felt that I had to take care of Mother and keep peace. This was more direct fact than fantasy. When I eventually left home, this blew my family apart, especially my parents' relationship. Subsequently my sister committed suicide and years later my parents were divorced. . . . My feelings burst forth in adolescence. I felt that I was a monster represented by breasts and menstrual periods and I had to starve my feelings to return to latency. This was the successful role where I could feel that I had a great family from the outside. My perception was that Father played the heavy role, and my mother needed protection from him. All this resulted in pain in my life that needed caring.

Life seemed out of control, without options to alter its course. Many reflected that anorexia was a way to stop time from moving forward. One subject remarked, " . . . getting sick was a way of telling people how terribly bad I was feeling, so that people would take me seriously."

All of the subjects reported that they became ill around the time of one or more of the following life events: school transitions (e.g., junior high to high school, move to college), a loss of friends or separation from family, or a troubling experience with love or sex. These milestones underscore how ill equipped the subject was to negotiate adolescence (Crisp, 1983b), separate from an ambivalently held object, or contend with sexuality (Bemporad and Ratey, 1985).

Experiences in Therapy

About 90% of the group rated some professional help as among the five most helpful and five most harmful experiences related to recovery. The expressed risks and benefits of each modality will be briefly reviewed.

Individual Psychotherapy. Although individual psychotherapy was by far the highest rated of all treatments, it was also viewed as potentially the most destructive. Most subjects had two or more courses of outpatient psychotherapy in addition to individual work they did while hospitalized, so we could readily compare therapeutic interventions.

Ideal qualities of the therapist include honesty, consistency, reliability, and flexibility. He/she should be nonjudgmental, trustworthy, and convey respect and warmth for the patient. The therapist should be very active, firm yet empathic, and confrontative when necessary. According to the subjects, it is important to depart from the technically neutral position and provide explanations about the eating disorder, coaching, and encouragement. The patients uniformly reacted negatively to inexplicit goals, inactivity, silences, and formality. They were anxious about recapitulating family dynamics, by being controlled with perceived hidden agendas and inexplicit rules, and exploited by an adult's narcissistic needs. Hence, they responded favorably to an open validation of who they really are and above all the therapist's facilitating better understanding of themselves and their family:

> I feel as though I was raised again from infancy, building a sense of myself. The therapy also gave me support that was confidential and separate from my family. He has been consistently supportive though never very directed or affected by my craziness. I didn't worry about hurting him.

The theme of both therapist and patient tolerating feelings, particularly anger, was extraordinarily important in therapy. The subjects pointed out that therapy helped to introduce them to feelings, to learn why they felt guilty, and to realize that anger cannot destroy a meaningful person. They emphatically stated that a serious error in psychotherapy is to blame parents excessively. A major task is to stop idealizing and forgive the mother:

> My first therapist hurt me because he refused to speak with my parents or deal with them. He tried to portray my parents as the enemy and painted

my mother as a demon. This was extremely harmful. Dr. T. told me I would leave therapy thinking of my mother as a friend. This was a great gift. Dr. T. worked hard to help me work through my feelings about my mother. She made it clear that my mother was a victim of her own circumstances and this helped me eventually forgive her and accept her without feeling oppressed. I also felt I was able to do this because I knew Dr. T. respected and admired me . . . she was down to earth, open and laughed at my jokes.

Effective psychotherapy permits risk taking both in the session and outside in relationships. The subjects found it valuable to receive coaching on how to interact with others. They noted that a skillful therapist can convey such instructions based on an empathic understanding of the patient and not on stock formulas. Good therapy increases self-confidence and trust in one's own feelings and ideas. This, in turn, facilitates separation from the family. Therapy becomes an important proving ground to test new ways of relating. To this extent, therapists need to be aware of the real relationship in addition to the transference and refrain from excessively controlling the patient:

Somebody looked me straight in the face, straight at my anorexia nervosa with me. I had the loving support from my fiance and support from my therapist. It's not what he did, it's what he is. He is not hesitant, he's confident, he listens. He was never judgmental. He saw me as a healthy person and always addressed that part of me. He addressed my strength and my healthy side and he did not let me be sick. Other doctors were afraid of my anorexia nervosa and never talked directly about it. He called me daily after my divorce, gave me his number on vacation; however, he did not baby me. He treated me as an adult. We could argue and I was terrified by my dependence on him. He never forced me to eat. He said you'll eat when you're ready. This was very important to me.

Therapists treating anorexics must have a solid working knowledge of eating disorders. Bruch (1982) feels explaining the course, dynamics, and complications of anorexia nervosa is most reassuring to patients. The subjects concur with this. However, they warn against inflexible adherence to one's own theory, a stance that impairs listening and understanding the patient as a unique individual. Moreover, imposing a theoretical structure on a patient repeats the experience of parents' dictating covertly or explicitly how to appear, feel, and think. The patient, in turn, relies on compliance gives the therapist exactly what he/she wants. Many anorexics are very well read; and, once they know where a therapist stands ideologically, will become "perfect patients." One subject in traditional psychoanalytic psychotherapy for seven years commented:

> . . . the blank expression was harmful. I was very concerned with doing it well, bringing in the right dreams, pleasing him, agreeing with the right interpretation.

In the same view, another subject reports:

> It was important and helpful for me to understand what I wanted and not to please others, to realize my motivations, my incredible set of rules, and thus to be able to accept myself.

Group Therapy and Self-Help Groups. Approximately half of the subjects had some experience in group therapy, which was evenly divided between formal group therapy and self-help groups. In general, group work was viewed as somewhat helpful. A common advantage of this modality was in establishing a forum for gaining the support and understanding of others struggling with the same issues and feelings. Yet bringing together a group of women with anorexia nervosa has its dangers. Many subjects felt the groups were too focused on food and dieting and allowed learning "bad habits" such as vomiting or ways to deceive physicians, like water loading before weight measurements. Some felt uneasy "comparing myself to other skeletons," envying the sicker members, and competing for the role of most impaired. This was especially worrisome in self-help groups without professional therapists as leaders to thwart such counterproductive, divisive behavior.

A few subjects felt safer in a group setting, finding it easier to identify feelings and use the support of the group to own them without guilt, fear, or shame. This was particularly true for subjects who were developmentally arrested before consolidating trust. These subjects, unable to integrate their own hostility and aggression utilized splitting, projection, and projective identification as core defenses. Such individuals with borderline traits (Kernberg, 1975) were plagued by omnipotent, magical thinking, terrified of the destructive power of their rage, threatened by its projection out into the world, and were ridden by unmodulated, primitive guilt. Although these women felt unworthy taking up the group's time, they found it safer than individual psychotherapy:

Feelings about self are especially terrifying in a one-to-one relationship. I feel powerful, as if I could destroy the therapist and me at the same time. With others I can reflect on feelings and it's less scary.

For patients like this, the combination of individual and group therapy was beneficial.

Family Therapy. Only a third of the group was exposed to family therapy and most often just during hospitalizations. Family therapy had mixed reviews. Those rating it harmful were bothered by an encouragement of ventilating anger without attempts to resolve conflict. "It didn't solve anything," one former anorexic reports, "it just rehashed the past. Sometimes we said hurtful things; we recognized that change was needed but no one was willing to change for me. It was entirely up to me to change how I saw and dealt with my family." Once a symptom bearer was brought to treatment she was faced with a seemingly insoluble conflict: if she chose the direction of health, engaging in family therapy to expose conflicts and alter relationships, such action would violate family loyalty and kindle hope of separation, for which she and her parents were unprepared. Threatened with dislodging a rigid, defensive though vulnerable family system, members colluded to resist therapeutic efforts. High functioning professional families are among the most difficult to treat and require experience and skill to prevent clinical errors:

Our therapist was totally inducted in the sick system. The problem was never redefined. In two years she never got my parents to deal with their issues and the kids to deal with theirs. Bad family therapy made individual therapy twice as hard. The therapist never disempowered my parents with regard to food, and she never took the focus off me, explained about my being a symptom bearer, even if it made my parents angry. She was sucked into my mother's control and little work was done.

In other hands, family therapy was invaluable, enabling members to be more open, and aware of each other's feelings. It could promote insight, "making my family see that events in my childhood had very much affected me in ways they weren't aware of," or it could help resolve core ambivalence in relationships. This is no easy task in families where pre-Oedipal conflicts predominate. Healing splitting, interpreting reaction formation, uncovering ruthless narcissistic needs and the bitter disappointments in not having them satisfied, and ameliorating primitive guilt require

. . . a gift: she (therapist) conveyed a lot of respect for each one of us to feel better about ourselves. This therapy enabled the family to bring out conflicts in a safe setting. What was most helpful was to learn that everyone and no one was to blame and to learn that in spite of our anger, mistakes, and hurt, we loved one another very deeply, and to discover that anger, mistakes, and hurt can coexist with love.

Prescribed Medication. Five subjects were prescribed medication during their illness. No one found them helpful in alleviating symptoms of anorexia nervosa per se; however, they were useful for the relief of anxiety, depression, and insomnia. In this respect, says one subject, "medications had a normalizing effect and allowed me to deal more effectively with my eating disorder."

On the other hand, medications were viewed as dangerous. They threatened to "take control and turn me into something else" and "led me to believe I couldn't do it on my own." Besides interfering with the perceived locus of control, drugs caused considerable adverse effects in the emaciated women, such as confusion, dizziness, constipation, memory loss, and fatigue. They also became potential sources of suicidal gestures. Finally, medications were taken, in part, as an alternative to the painful struggles in psychotherapy: "Medications enabled me to eat without anxiety or depression, but getting off them I hadn't learned anything about how to handle those nagging drives to lose weight in the real world."

Hospitalization. Most anorexics, terrified of relinquishing control, enter the hospital under duress. In our clinical experience, hospitalization is usually met by the patient initially with active or passive resistance, indignation, deceptiveness, emotional constriction, cold indifference, or outright hostility. Inpatient treatment, though usually successful in achieving weight gain, is notoriously difficult both for the patients and staff. We were surprised to find that the subjects, although expressing some strong negative reactions, rated hospitalization as helpful and at times clearly life saving. Three-quarters of the group were hospitalized and over a third had multiple admissions.

On the negative side, many patients objected to the hair-splitting emphasis on weight gain and the demeaning aspects of behavior therapy. They felt devalued, humiliated, and condemned being constantly watched. It was particularly trying when staff had deficient empathic understanding of their problem. Finally, many complained that inadequate attention was given to the transition out of hospital, making the readjustment to home and/or school difficult:

> In some ways the hospital was valuable, providing a space to be sick, but it also defeated the root problems of anorexia, that is, the need to form a self, which is in self-control, aware of my needs and not controlled. I had been controlled all my life, which led to an inability to take care of myself. In the hospital, it was safe to eat, but I was totally aware that I could re-lose the weight when discharged. It focused on my illness and not a family problem. Behavior modification is a joke because anorectics are too smart. They do what they want to do and what they need to do to get out. No one can make you get better.

Most subjects, despite their overt defiance and anxiety, felt relieved that someone was taking over, structuring their world, and making decisions for them, particularly about food. Although in one respect, medical and behavioral monitoring felt intrusive, it was nevertheless perceived as an act of caring. The hospital presented an assurance of safety, a refuge from home, school, and friends. It forced them to confront their problems and with the support from staff and especially peers, facilitated open expression of their fears of food and being fat. The hospital demonstrated how to value and care for themselves.

Experiences Outside Therapy

Life experiences were seen in much the same light as therapy related experiences: high risk, high yield – potentially destructive, confirming the fragility of the self and need for the defensive anorexic stance, but at the same time potentially rewarding, offering opportunities for personal growth and healing old wounds. About 90% of subjects rated some nontherapy experience as among the five most helpful and five most harmful experiences related to recovery. Former anorexics were telling us two things: experiences outside therapy are just as important as experiences in therapy in the process of recovery, and engagement in either realm requires extreme caution. Areas that were deemed important include self-initiated action/personal experience of self, interpersonal relationships, family relationships, and job or school experiences.

We now might turn to the concept of "spontaneous recovery"

and generate a hypothesis: "Spontaneous recovery" is not simply dependent on the natural history of anorexia nervosa, but rather on meaningful relationships and experiences in life that have therapeutic impact. Although this is not terribly surprising, it may have profound implications for the conduct of therapy with anorexics. As therapists, too often we place such a high premium on the process of our work that we forget or minimize the therapeutic value of experiences in daily life. Perhaps as Goodsitt (1985) advises, the therapist should compensate for deficits in the self by offering himself as a self object or transitional object, and actively teach, coach, and encourage the patient to participate in growth promoting life experiences.

Self-Initiated Action/Personal Experience of Self

Oppressed with paralyzing ineffectiveness (Bruch, 1982), anorexics experience a self-initiated action as truly liberating. Most of our subjects reported that they recalled rebellious acts or decisions not to do something expected of one, such as leaving school or refusing treatment recommendations, pivotal therapeutic experiences. As such, these decisions instilled a sense of power, effectiveness, dignity, and independence. Interestingly, although all subjects described the road to recovery as a painfully slow process, the majority had a common experience: they vividly remembered a specific occasion on which they told themselves, "I am bored with this," or "I am sick of this." They saw the turning point experientially as making a personal decision to change and give up the anorexia as an act of will, once it felt sufficiently ego-dystonic. The inner meaning of this intrapsychic event was that they experienced their change as personal, self-determined, and independent of others' decisions, advice, or feelings.

The process of recovery was akin to a psychological rebirth. It necessitated getting to know themselves better. Many found that self-understanding was enhanced by talking to themselves, particularly about their feeling states, desires, and body image. A few recalled the value of talking to themselves in front of a mirror. Another instrument for self-reflection was keeping a diary and reading it over and over again. These behaviors may be understood as transitional phenomena, described by Winnicott (1958), in which the talking or writing becomes a means of self-soothing, utilizing illusion to combat a pervasive sense of aloneness. Virtually all the subjects had meaningful transitional objects during their illness and recovery. Once feelings could be identified and acknowledged, it became immensely important to express them to others. The inner experience of psychological rebirth was described as "finding an identity other than one wrapped up in anorexia nervosa, and using opportunities in my life to test and experiment with what I learned about myself."

Interpersonal Relationships. A critical step in recovery is taking the risk of exposing oneself to others. As one former anorexic described, "I could finally accept myself, when friends got to see me as I really was, without acting, and that meant seeing all sides of me, the good and the bad." It takes great courage for an anorexic patient to make herself vulnerable by asking help from friends. Even more valuable is falling in love with a man. About a third of our group told us that a landmark event was developing an intimate relationship. Both the friendship and the sex helped them not to be ashamed of one's body and to take pleasure in it:

> My boyfriend has opened me up sexually, made me confident. We walk together, we work together, and we learn together. It took four to six months to be naked in the daylight and feel comfortable with him.

> It was important for my recovery to have a relationship with a man. I did not have many intimate relationships with men and those relationships I did have with men were very conflicted, for example my father and brother. My boyfriend had very strong positive feelings for me. We ate meals together. He really helped turn me around. I asked him if I were too skinny and he said "yes" directly and could tell me openly how I looked and how it made him feel. . . . Sex was liberating. He would see my body and not be critical. He wasn't modest or ashamed of his body. He allowed give and take and nurturance. This balance was very important. I became in touch with my feelings of love and warmth and felt I deserved them in return. He helped me relax and experience the pleasure of my body.

Intimate relationships are not without their liabilities. As noted previously, a number of women attributed the onset of their anorexia nervosa to a troubling experience in love. One has to be ready for sexual involvement:

> It was a frightening experience to see another person go away. I was distrustful, I lost my self-worth, I felt weak. Staying thin, one can't think straight. Lack of help from friends is very harmful. A sexual relationship is very harmful if one is not ready for it. It is a "should." I became frigid in

my first year, he couldn't penetrate me. Sex was horrible. I didn't want to be a sexual woman, I wanted to be held like a little girl.

Family Relationships. All of our subjects pointed to family relationships as a cause of their illness. They often found help from family harmful. Over half felt that being away from family was extremely helpful. This group also considered the understanding of family dynamics, made possible by separation, a vital part of recovery. Families were generally not seen as health promoting. Negative influences included derogatory remarks about not eating, the inability to understand the meaning of the illness, lack of time to be involved, avoidance of conflict, persistence in "controlling me and telling me what I feel and what I should do," and overprotection. Some felt that the experience of "being able to make a decision disapproved of by my parents, and seeing that we can all tolerate and accept it" was helpful. In many cases, after symptoms of anorexia abated, family relations improved. This took one of two routes: In families where significant therapeutic work was accomplished, relationships improved, marked by open, honest communication and expression of feeling; in families resistant to change, the anorexics eventually gave up longings for idealized parent figures and came to terms with who their parents really were, accepting their limitations.

Job or School Experience. These subjects uniformly agreed that productivity in work or school was a valuable asset. These activities seemed to help by instilling feelings of power, effectiveness, achievement, and satisfaction as opposed to attaining similar feelings by focusing on food restriction and weight reduction. Work was only a problem when the anorexics were confronted in some way about their weight. Some lost jobs because of their appearance. Others were hurt by being labeled and stigmatized by their eating disorders and expended considerable energy, concern, and anxiety concealing past and current problems.

Features Hardest to Change

Although the behavioral eating patterns were difficult to overcome, especially the eating disorder as a "relief valve" and "coping mechanism," most of our subjects felt compulsions and impulses were far easier to control than perceptions and obsessional thinking. Long after eating was relatively normal, intrusive, obsessive thoughts about food and weight persisted, often determining how one felt the rest of the day. The eating behavior most refractory to change was eating in social situations. Most former anorexics could proudly recall milestones such as going out for pizza and beer with friends and feeling comfortable. Of the perceptual abnormalities, the most recalcitrant was distortion of body image:

> I still don't have a good body image. It took a very long time after recovering from anorexia nervosa to realize what I really looked like. Even now I stare at my old pictures and I can't see anything. The fear of going from 70 to 200 pounds is very hard to change. The first bite is the hardest. If you start, it feels like you will never stop.

Many reported that body image was the last thing to change and there still are residual distortions. This quotation also typifies the difficulty in altering the anorexic dichotomous all-or-nothing thinking. The tendency to see things in extremes — fat or thin, good or bad, smart or dumb, lazy or active, loved or hated, continues for quite some time after weight gain.

Self-devaluation, envy, guilt, and compensatory drive for perfection also last long after weight restoration:

> I feel my mind and I are partners now. Formerly we were enemies. The hardest thing to change is to stop your mind from the anorectic thought process. Even if it does not focus on weight and food there was the perpetual comparing myself with others, feeling inadequate, ugly, not good enough or smart enough. Low self-esteem is very difficult to change. It took a long time to accept myself including my limitations and not condemn myself as much. Finally, I could take away all the nagging "shoulds" in my life.

What Was Lost by Giving Up Anorexia Nervosa

However maladaptive, anorexia nervosa serves an essential defensive function. At some point, for many of the reasons described previously, these women were able to relinquish their symptomatic behavior, perception, and thought process. We were curious what repercussions this gradual but radical change had on a person's intrapsychic equilibrium, and so we posed the questions: "What did you lose by giving up your anorexia nervosa? What took its place?"

Initially, many subjects tended to feel a loss of self-respect by "giving in," as if their motivation to get well was a defeat and betrayal of themselves. Moreover, they felt increasingly afraid of rejection. It felt like losing "protective armor" that helped "avoid growing up, being independent, taking care of oneself, and making one's own decisions." A prominent theme was a sense at first of losing specialness, only to regain it in other healthier ways:

> I lost a specialness that I thought it gave me. I was different from everyone else. Now I know that I'm somebody who's overcome it, which not everybody does.

> Self acceptance took its place. I lost my rigid obsessiveness, my robot-type existence. I lost my impatience. I feel safer now. I can believe in my own judgment now and not theirs. People used to take advantage of me. Not anymore. I thought by controlling food, I could control my life concretely, but this was really not the case. Being skinny I felt special. Now it's not being skinny that I feel special. I still feel different from others, but in some positive sense.

These questions, we are sure, would be much more difficult to answer by ill anorexics in the midst of change. Looking back, most former anorexics see their losses as dysfunctional, ego dystonic states such as misery, depression, obsessiveness, feeling driven, inability to relax, excessive guilt, and impatience. From their current vantage point, they experienced a wealth of positive traits taking its place: feelings, an ability to have fun, positive self-regard, self-respect in areas other than denial and deprivation, trusting one's own capabilities, and having a sense of identity other than anorexia nervosa.

> I lost nothing. What took its place? Curiosity, laughter, joy, adventure, opening my eyes to what there is and experiencing my feelings.

> I didn't have much to lose. What I had to lose was misery and a negative way of thinking and many tears. Nothing was right. I felt driven by anorexia nervosa, slowed down. What took its place? Seeing, hearing, tasting things, mental acuity. This was never present. I can feel now. I miss people now and I enjoy being with them.

> I gave up being powerful. I gave up rituals and magic. I gave up laxatives. I gave up my constant stomach problems. I gave up my mother as the perfect mother and being symbiotic with her. Would she survive if we separated? What took its place? I took its place.

The Question of Complete Recovery

Half of our subjects believe people fully recover from anorexia nervosa; half disagree, making an analogy to alcoholism — a life-long illness that can be progressively controlled albeit with less and less effort. Although the two groups differed on their ultimate answer to the question of complete recovery, there was uniform agreement that recovering is a lengthy, slow process and they are left with certain remnants of the disorder. All retain excessive concerns about food and weight, but no longer feel consumed by them. Other common residual features include some fragility in self-esteem, sensitivity to rejection and a tendency under pressure, when things go wrong or when angry at parents, to return to old ways of thinking:

> It really is like alcoholism — a process of recovering. I keep it in check one day at a time. One of the hardest things was throwing away my small clothes. My doctor says anorexia nervosa just goes away. No, it doesn't. It's not on the surface much of the time, but one difficult day at the job or with my family, I tend to find myself going back to the thought processes of anorexia, because I used to think this was safe.

Recovery for all former patients means self-acceptance, "knowing who you are, trusting your feelings and judgment, getting rid of rigid 'shoulds' and rules, all resulting in feeling free, safe, and in control." A pivotal hallmark of change is a sense of "lightening up" and a new found ability to play:

> I'm comfortable now, not driven. I still have conflicts with my mother, but that's okay. I can play now for the first time. I can laugh. I enjoy eating. I eat more than my fiance and I eat like a kid. I can go into a crowd and I'm not afraid to try new things. It's a process of recovering really. Probably I'll always watch what I'll eat, but which woman doesn't? It's very unlikely that I'll go back. What's left? Life, living. I still get cold, I'm still sensitive to meds and some foods give me discomfort. What's left? I'm a great cook. Some perfectionism is also left. I'm more relaxed now. What's left? Being human; it's easier than sainthood.

A crucial element in the process of recovering was being able to tolerate anger and resentment, particularly toward the mother, live more comfortably with ambivalence and subsequently not feel as oppressed by guilt:

I'm still obsessed with my stomach and food, but it has changed in degree. It doesn't rule my life. I do count calories in my head and I'm still concerned but I'm *not* afraid of being fat. Fear is losing control. As a person I feel grounded in my sense of self. Yes, people absolutely recover in the sense that you can stop starving, hating yourself, loathing yourself. It's possible because I had to realize that my mother was so important that I became miniscule. It wasn't important if I lived or died. If I could have been perfect, everything would have been okay. If not perfect, I hated myself and did not deserve to eat. The process of recovering is a process of liking oneself again. This can be done through therapeutic or real relationships, through mutual respect, boundaries and a new relationship with my parents. Right now I have a fine relationship with them. My mother has changed since I stopped trying to change her. That's very important. I'm not trying to buy into her garbage anymore and I know my own limits. The result of all this is making my own choices, like my boyfriend. This was the primary way of separating from my family. Although they disapproved since he is of another race, I followed my heart.

Advice to Others Suffering from Anorexia Nervosa

The question of advice was addressed first by emphasizing a deep conflict for the anorexic. When ill, nothing anyone can say or do will help. In fact, the more someone tries, the more the anorexic resists: "You will only do it when you are ready." Actually, beyond this hurdle, advice was rather uniform and straightforward. Despite a reluctance to admit it, an anorexic desperately needs another person who relates to her honestly, encouraging expression of feelings and exploring together who she is. The key is the anorexic's relinquishing her defensive battle cry "Let me be!" (Crisp, 1983b).

As much as it seems terrifying not to be skinny, instead of spending so much time on yourself and your anorexic symptoms and cutting yourself off from others, you must learn to reach out. There is a tremendous amount of nurturance and caring if you can let it happen and take the risk of trusting others with what you feel. The rituals actually cut this off. You need to work with someone you trust. *Don't do it alone!* You need another's perception to show you that yours is distorted. Looks are not as important as what you feel. Increasing awareness of one's thoughts and feelings gives a person increased courage about themselves, about getting well. You need to deal with yourself as you really are and not what you aim to be. Self-acceptance is important. It can be yours more naturally. One needs to be honest. It feels like I've gone straight. The secrecy is gone. People don't know who you really are when you're anorexic, in part because you don't know who you are.

SUMMARY

The women who participated in this study told us much about their experience of change and recovery from anorexia nervosa. The evolution from illness to health was much like the Velveteen Rabbit's becoming REAL. When ill, the anorexic has no idea what it is like to be a real person with a cohesive sense of self, known and loved by others for herself. Unable to accurately identify and express feelings, and alienated from meaningful relationships, the anorexic pursues a mechanical existence based on compliance and distorted perceptions of bodily functions. Indeed, she does not feel REAL. The process of recovering from anorexia nervosa is the process of becoming a person. We learned that the essential therapeutic agent for this lengthy change is establishment of a relationship — either with a therapist or someone in everyday life. Through the medium of being empathically understood by another person, the anorexic begins to learn who she is. With the sense that someone is really with her, she can begin to unravel her maladaptive, self-destructive defenses, which served to protect her from her feelings and impulses and isolate her from the world.

We conclude that the notion of "spontaneous recovery" may be misleading. The process of recovering from anorexia nervosa requires the resolution of pathological object relations, and this can only be accomplished in the context of a human relationship. Although some anorexic defensive structure remains, these women are able to engage in healthy adult relationships and activities with a secure sense of themselves.

References

Bassoe, H. H., and Eskeland, I. (1982), A prospective study of 133 patients with anorexia nervosa, *Acta Psychiatria Scandinavica, 65*, 127–133.

Bemporad, J. R., and Ratey, J. (1985), Intensive psychotherapy of former anorexic individuals, *Am. J. Psychother., 39*, 454–465.

Bruch, H. (1973), *Eating Disorders: Obesity, Anorexia Nervosa, and the Person Within*, Basic Books, New York.

Bruch, H. (1982), Anorexia nervosa: Therapy and theory, *Am. J. Psychiatry, 139*, 1531–1538.

Crisp, A. H. (1983a), Treatment and outcome in anorexia nervosa, in R. K. Goodstein (Ed.), *Eating and Weight Disorders: Advances in Treatment and Research*, Springer, New York.

Crisp, A. H. (1983b), *Anorexia Nervosa: Let Me Be*, Grune & Stratton, New York.

Dally, P. J. (1969), *Anorexia Nervosa*, Grune and Stratton, New York.

Garfinkel, P. E., and Garner, D. M. (1982), Prognosis, in *Anorexia Nervosa: A Multidimensional Perspective*, Brunner/Mazel, New York.

Garner, D. M., Olmstead, M. P., and Polivy, J. (1983), Eating Disorders Inventory, Psychological Assessment Resources, Inc., Toronto.

Geist, R. A. (1985), Therapeutic dilemmas in the treatment of anorexia nervosa: A self-psychological perspective, in S. W. Emmett (Ed.), *Theory and Treatment of Anorexia Nervosa and Bulimia: Biomedical, Sociocultural and Psychological Perspectives*, Brunner/Mazel, New York, pp. 268–288.

Goodsitt, A. (1983), Self-regulatory disturbances in eating disorders, *Int. J. Eating Disorders, 1*, 70–76.

Goodsitt, A. (1985), Self psychology in the treatment of anorexia nervosa, in D. M. Garner and P. E. Garfinkel (Eds.), *Handbook of Psychotherapy for Anorexia Nervosa and Bulimia*, Guilford Press, New York, pp. 55–82.

Gordon, C., Beresin, E. V., and Herzog, D. B. (1989), The parents' relationship and child's illness in anorexia nervosa. *J. Am. Acad. Psychoanal., 17*, 29–42.

Hall, A., Slim, E., Hawker, F., and Salmond, C. (1984), Anorexia nervosa: Long-term outcome in 50 female patients, *Br. J. Psychiatry, 145*, 407–413.

Hsu, L. K. G. (1980), Outcome of anorexia nervosa, *Arch. Gen. Psychiatry, 37*, 1041–1046.

Hsu, L. K. G., and Crisp, A. H. (1980), The Crown-Crisp Experimental Index (CCEI) profile in anorexia nervosa, *Br. J. Psychiatry, 136*, 567–573.

Hsu, L. K. G., Crisp, A. H., and Harding, B. (1979), Outcome of anorexia nervosa, *Lancet, 1*, 61–65.

Johnson, C., and Connors, M. E. (1987), *The Etiology and Treatment of Bulimia Nervosa*, Basic Books, New York.

Kernberg, O. (1980), Melanie Klein, in H. I. Kaplan, A. M. Freedman, and B. J. Sadock, (Eds.), *Comprehensive Textbook of Psychiatry*, William and Wilkins, Baltimore, pp. 802–833.

Kernberg, O. (1975), *Borderline Conditions and Pathological Narcissism*, Jason Aronson, New York.

Masterson, S. F. (1977), Primary anorexia nervosa in the borderline adolescent — an object relations view, in P. Harticollis (Ed.), *Borderline Personality Disorders*, International Universities Press, New York.

Minuchin, S., Rosman, B. L., and Baker, L. (1978), *Psychomatic Families*, Harvard University Press, Cambridge.

Morgan, H. G., Purgold, J., and Welbourne, J. (1983), Management and outcome in anorexia nervosa: A standardized prognostic study, *Br. J. Psychiatry, 143*, 282–287.

Morgan, H. G., and Russell, G. F. M. (1975), Value of family background and clinical features as predictors of long-term outcome in anorexia nervosa: Four year follow-up study of 41 patients, *Psychol. Med., 5*, 355–371.

Niskanen, P., Jaaskelainen, J., and Achte, K. (1974), Anorexia nervosa: Treatment results and prognosis, *Psychiatria Fennica*, 257–263.

Nussbaum, M., Shanker, R., Baird, D., and Saravay, S. (1985), Follow-up investigation in patients with anorexia nervosa, *J. Pediatrics, 106*, 835–840.

Palazzoli, M. S. (1978), *Self-Starvation*, Jason Aronson, New York.

Piazza, E., Piazza, N., and Rollins, N. M. (1980), Anorexia nervosa: Controversial aspects of therapy, *Comp. Psychiatry, 21*, 177–189.

Rizzuto, A. M. (1985), Eating and monsters: A psychological view of bulimarexia, in S. W. Emmett (Ed.), *Theory and Treatment of Anorexia Nervosa: Biomedical, Sociocultural and Psychological Perspectives*, Brunner/Mazel, New York, pp. 194–210.

Rizzuto, A. M., Peterson, R. K., and Reed, M. (1981), The pathological sense of self in anorexia nervosa, *Psychiatric Clinics of North America, 4*, 471–487.

Rollins, N., and Blackwell, A. (1968), The treatment of anorexia nervosa in children and adolescents: Stage 1, *J. Child Psychol. Psychiat., 9*, 81–91.

Rollins, N., and Piazza, E. (1981), Anorexia nervosa: A quantitative approach to follow-up, *J. Am. Acad. Child Psychiatry, 20*, 167–183.

Schwartz, D. M., and Thompson, M. G. (1981), Do anorectics get well? Current research and future needs, *Am. J. Psychiatry, 138*, 319–323.

Sours, J. A. (1980), *Starving to Death in a Sea of Objects*, Jason Aronson, New York.

Stonehill, E., and Crisp, A. H. (1977), Psychoneurotic characteristics of patients with anorexia nervosa before and after treatment and at follow-up 4–7 years late, *J. Psychosom. Res., 21*, 189–193.

Sugarman, A., and Kurash, C. (1982), The body as transitional object in bulimia, *Int. J. Eating Disorders, 1*, 57–67.

Swift, W. J:, and Letven, R. (1984), Bulimia and the basic fault: A psychoanalytic interpretation of the binge-vomiting syndrome, *J. Am. Acad. Child Psychiatry, 23*, 489–497.

Weissman, M. M., and Bothwell, S. (1976), Assessment of social adjustment by patient self-report, *Arch. Gen. Psychiatry, 33*, 1111–1115.

Weissman, M. M., Prusoff, B. A., et al. (1978), Social adjustment by self report in a community sample and in psychiatric outpatients, *J. Nerv. Ment. Dis., 166*, 317–326.

Williams, M. (1975), *The Velveteen Rabbit or How Toys Become Real*, Avon Books, New York.

Winnicott, D. W. (1958), Transitional objects and transitional phenomena, in *Through Pediatrics to Psychoanalysis*, Basic Books, New York, pp. 229–242.

Yager, J., Landsverk, J., and Edelstein, C. K. (1987), A 20-month follow-up study of 628 women with eating disorders, I: Course and severity, *Am. J. Psychiatry, 144*, 1172–1177.

Child Psychiatry Service, ACC-625
Massachusetts General Hospital
15 Parkman Street
Boston, MA 02114

BULIMIA: THE CONSTRUCTION
OF A SYMPTOM

PAUL HAMBURG, M.D.

The purpose of this paper is to explore a psychiatric symptom: bulimia. A natural departure point is to consider the usual meaning of a symptom in medicine. Symptoms belong to the realm of semiology; they are signs that suggest a mystery. Symptoms have a painful manifest reality. They may also contain a latent reality that explains the patient's discomfort. The symptom is necessarily ambiguous. Chest pain may tell a story of coronary occlusion, or it may not. Headache may reveal the tension of overwork, or it may disclose a brain tumor. This latency of meaning has the quality of a clue, a signpost along our way of inquiry. Signs have several common characteristics, including polysemy (the generation of multiple strands of meaning) and ambiguity. Even as they represent an aspect of reality, they do so without total equivalence, inevitably adding something here, transforming something else there. Signs generate meaning beyond representation, by virtue of their nonequivalence and ambiguity. Contained within the additions and subtactions of the sign are traces of other significant meanings.

We can welcome symptoms as clues to an underlying process. Naturally we are first impressed by the pain of the symptom itself, yet we are also confronted by uncertainty, mystery, and the possibility of many meanings. This is particularly the case for psychiatric symptoms, if we regard them as pathways to the unconscious. Freud (1926/1959) describes the synthetic quality of symptoms "which once stood for a restriction of the ego (and) come to represent satisfactions as well." He also notes the "extremely restricted ego" that is the consequence of symptom formation. The psychiatric symptom is at once a source of distress to the patient, a complex assortment of unconscious meaning, a form of communication, and a cause for our own discomfort as we seek to unravel its interweavings.

Bulimia is a ritually repetitive sequence of acts, which begin

From the Eating Disorders Unit and General Psychiatry Practice, Massachusetts General Hospital.

with a dysphoric feeling-state that anticipates a binge. There follow preparations for binging and then the orgiastic consumption of a very large quantity of food. After a moment of suspension in fullness, the terrible fear of becoming fat and the guilt of having yielded to desire lead to a forceful purge or a deliberate restriction of further eating. The episode ends in a feeling-state that often mixes relief and shame. As witnesses to this ritual we should be intrigued by the multiple clues it suggests to us, themes of orality, anality, consumption, the body ego, control, desire, humiliation, and so forth. The richness of these themes is striking. Depending on our theoretical bias, we might privilege one theme or another and search for the single, best, all-encompassing interpretation of the symptom-sign. We might focus on the dysphoria produced by the symptom, call it a disease, and crusade against it as though its other meanings were irrelevant. We might select the theme of oral fixation, and try to understand the bulimic's world in terms of emptiness, need, greed, taking-in, fullness, and attempts to control the narcissistic supply network by narrowing all desire to the desire for food. We might speculate about the culture of narcissism, and see the bulimic symptom as a metaphor for a social order whose material values have subverted the fulfillment of real human needs. There are a host of other possibilities, each departing from one theme contained in the complex metaphor that is the symptom.

The quest for a solitary underlying meaning is only one approach to the problem. It assumes that the mystery has one solution, one basic hidden truth, and narrows the science of interpretation to an unveiling of this basic truth. Sometimes this approach makes sense in the diagnostic interpretation of medical symptoms and signs. Unfortunately, the search for an ultimate meaning denies the complexity of the psychiatric symptom. In confronting the inevitable competition of different contexts and interpretations we need to ask whether the function of a symptom might not be precisely to weave together diverse contexts into a single metaphorical fabric. By deferring the search for one correct interpretation and instead examining the relationship among several meanings of a symptom we might learn more about the symptom's capacity to integrate aspects of the patient's world. The layering of meanings may be an essential aspect of the symptom-sign, only obscured by our own need for simplification, explanation, and certainty. If the goal shifts from a search for the single true meaning of the symptom to a description of multiple meanings and contexts, the task becomes finding a way to look at a complex phenomenon without succumbing to a sense of chaos. The exploration of a hierarchy of interpretive possibilities by deferring the search for ultimate explanations is part of an analytic method developed by Jacques Derrida as a tool of literary-philosophical criticism, called deconstruction (Derrida, 1978). Much of this method is derived from a radical consideration of signs and their relationship to what they signify. This paper seeks to extend the methods of deconstructive analysis to the understanding of a psychiatric symptom.*

Symptoms can be seen as complex acts of communication. If the symptom is a message, then we can ask to whom it is addressed. Messages may appear to have specific destinations; more typically they spread their meaning transferentially in multiple directions. If we see the symptom as a homeostatic message, then its biologic addressee may be opiate receptors in the limbic system. If we see the symptom as an act of intrapsychic communication, then its unconscious destination lies within the self. In this context, the bulimic cements a self in danger of fragmenting. If we see the symptom as an act of interpersonal communication, then food takes the place of a person and the ritual of bulimia may contain complex metaphors of relationship. If we see the symptom as a statement in a family drama, then it might be an attempt to hold the center in a troubled family amidst double threats of alienation and enmeshment. If we see the symptom as cultural communication, then it might represent a reductio-ad-absurdum of consumerism, where goods substitute for human needs and wanton waste fuels rituals of consumption. The symptom carries a message with all of these destinations, in the same way that its meanings link

*Deconstruction is an approach to interpretation that has its roots in psychoanalysis, structuralism, and phenomenology. From psychoanalysis it derives an active respect for the unconscious; from structuralism, a rigorous attention to the symbolic process; and from phenomenology, a probing concern for the language of human experience. Deconstruction does not strive to be a transcendental theory; instead, it inserts the interpretive process into the margins, spaces, and ambiguities of texts, questioning assumptions that permeate words, philosophical systems, and ordinary discourse. Deconstruction pays particular attention to the gaps between symbols and what they represent, opening seemingly slight divergences to reveal unexpected latent possibilities. It explores these differences by challenging the privileged centers of Western philosophic tradition: theocentrism (God as the center of meaning), phallocentrism (the masculine as the center of meaning), and logocentrism (the Word as the center of meaning). The application of deconstruction to the practice of psychoanalytic interpretation is an area of rich potential for future exploration.

multiple contexts. Perhaps the symptom's value to the patient arises from its capacity to communicate many meanings in many directions. Once again the challenge is to place these destinations of the symptom-message in perspective.

A symptom, then, is a clue to multiple contexts of communicated meaning. It reveals and conceals simultaneously. Our task is to explore hidden meanings while balancing the multiplicity of their implied contexts. This task requires a willingness to appreciate the symptom despite being unable to restrict the play of its meanings. We must maintain our respect for the complexity of the unconscious.

The etymology of "symptom" provides a reference point in our search for an understanding of the bulimic symptom. The Greek roots "sym" and "tom" mean falling-together. At one level we can contrast the formation of a symptom (falling-together) with disintegration (falling apart): the psychiatric symptom is an organizing phenomenon that limits a threatened fragmentation of the self even while causing its own measure of distress. Faced with a threat, the developing self experiences a fall; the creation of a symptom permits the preservation of a measure of integrity, as opposed to free-fall into chaos. The implication of this view is that the symptom arises in response to an impasse (developmental, psychological, biological) that threatens to disrupt the self. The symptom manifests the ongoing pain of that impasse, while significantly containing its psychological consequences. The bulimic symptom bears the marks of a pathological response—a fall—but it also serves to organize the self in a way that partially preserves its integrity. The symptom tells a dual story, of a fall and a recovery from falling.

A second implication of falling-together is that the formation of a psychiatric symptom has the effect of contracting the inner world. Bulimia forces a retreat from the social and interpersonal world to focus upon the body and its orifices. There is a loss of space in this falling-together, a collapse of a richer world into a smaller, poorer one. The body becomes a fortress to contain further collapse. The outer world of people and things becomes absorbed into the metaphoric language of food; it, too, has lost much of its diversity in the falling-together of symptom formation. This contraction is a striking aspect of the world bulimic patients describe to us.

A third implication of the symptom seen as falling-together is that of a collapse in mental structure, a developmental retreat that blends spaces, zones, and desires into a less differentiated amalgam. Although the elements of further development remain detectable in this amalgam, they seem to blend one into the other. The symptom represents a preservation of organization, but at a more primitive, condensed level. In this respect, the collapse of structure implied by the bulimic symptom can be described in three divergent but entwined metaphors: an oral world, an anal world, and a genital world.

Bulimia collapses experience into orality. In the oral world there is an economics of supply; an enormous vacuum lies deep within the body. Before the binge, there is an aching hunger, an emptiness coupled with the searching desire for fulfillment. The state of seeking is experienced as profoundly painful. At times this can be manifested in therapy by the power of a searching gaze that seeks to consume the therapist. It may take the form of uncontrollable shopping sprees, theft, acquiring useless things to fill up rooms and houses as well as stomach. Food is the magic drug that soothes excitement and relieves wanting. The world becomes a giant filling station whose supplies can obliterate the empty tension of desire. There is no measure of sufficiency: only excess. Points of view, personal qualities, gestures, and styles can also be consumed intact and incorporated in the personality. Displaying one's body surface for the desiring other makes the bulimic patient feel wanted, but only as the other person's next meal. Merging with the other, blending of selves, and feeling consumed by the other constitute an oral register of relationship.

Bulimia collapses experience into anality. In the anal world there is an economics of shame. Hunger is experienced as humiliating need; the food that was just consumed as a magic drug to fill an inner void becomes a poison as it enters the body: it must turn into vomit or diarrhea just so it should not instead turn into ugly fat. Affluent excess is thereby transformed into effluents. An associative chain links excess, fat, dirt, bodily defectiveness, ugliness, and the shamefulness of ever having wanted anything. In this anal world the only hope rests in the possibility of completely purging this awful badness. A burst of power, an assertion of control, and perhaps this humiliation can be overcome. After the purge, there remains a depleted, exhausted emptiness.

Bulimia collapses experience into genitality. In the genital world there is an economics of excitement; hunger is sexualized. The binge is eagerly anticipated, planned, and accomplished in a sensual frenzy. Its stimulation enlivens the deadness within, and affectively charges the entire body to overcome its emptiness and mitigate its aloneness. There is a rhythmic quality of this excitement that may be manifested in strenuous exercise and vigorous activity; the body comes to life in movement. The bulimic patient may stimulate the people around her, including the therapist; by arousing their excitement, she assures their concern for her. Excitement is a shiny envelope that preserves inner life.

In the sequence of actions that form the bulimic symptom, these three collapsed worlds are entwined through their failures. The oral world fails when food threatens to turn into badness even as it soothes and fills, and the bulimic ritual passes toward the anal world. The anal world also fails when the purge does not completely rid the self of badness. The bulimic patient turns to renewed stimulation or to food. The genital world fails when excitement becomes irritation. The bulimic patient then turns back to food to soothe her excitement. Other experiences enter the same registers of meaning. For example, the bulimic patient may describe an unwanted pregnancy and subsequent abortion in the same language as she describes her food binges and purges. She feels a desire to be filled up and to be held, to be excited and contained. With the knowledge of impregnation, she feels a mixture of fullness, humiliation, and the immediate need to be rid of this excess. The abortion comes as a profound relief, only to be followed by a lasting sense of shame, a recurrent feeling of even greater emptiness, the need to forget, and a wave of bulimic or sexual activity.

As a metaphor, the bulimic symptom interweaves diverse threads of meaning, borrowing from at least three systems of psychological economy to organize a retreat from the complexities of a more differentiated world. The symptom represents a collapse of a richer, more spacious structure and entails a significant loss of difference. This is true of any ritualization of experience. Rituals reduce play and space, even as they organize reality. For the bulimic, inner space feels like a cloacal cavity; it is enormous, empty, unfillable and its emptiness hurts. This cavity combines qualities that are mouthlike, alimentary, and womblike. The distortion in inner space is paralleled by a distortion of body form, with each small increment of flesh felt as a ponderous excess that depletes personal value. Cognitive differences are similarly collapsed, particularly as they relate to sensitive themes of desire, indulgence, being seen, and accommodating the needs of the other. Like any retreat into ritualized action, the symptom engenders a loss of spontaneity.

In deciding how to approach a symptom in psychotherapy, we need to be able to balance our respect for the architect with our compassion for the sufferer. In describing symptoms, Freud almost always added the word "Bildung" (Laplanche and Pontalis, 1973). The German "Bildung" has usually been translated into English and French as "formation," but it has a more elaborate meaning, one that implies construction, elaboration, informing, giving form, and substantiation. The Bildung of a symptom is a creative act of mental architecture. A therapeutic alliance must include a connection with the builder of symptoms that keep the patient's fall in the realm of falling-together rather than falling apart. The "deconstruction" of a symptom seeks to restore the complexity concealed in its construction.

What should be our psychotherapeutic relationship with the symptom? The symptom is a sufficient cause of suffering that it is often the principal reason a patient first solicits our help. The symptom is also an attempt to solve a psychological dilemma; this describes its creative aspect. The elaboration of metaphors, signs, and symptoms is part of the constructive-creative activity of the mind. Without the symptom, conditions might be worse.

One approach is to define the symptom as the disease. It is the enemy, so we must launch a battle. The symptom must be destroyed. This approach is flawed in several respects. It neglects the function of the symptom in maintaining psychological equilibrium. It also confirms the anal perspective of the bulimic's world: there is a badness within that must be purged. Therapy then becomes another repetition of the purging process, with its inevitable price of humiliation. Like the symptom, a purgative therapy may be partially successful to contain the patient's world, but does little to heal a fragmented self. In fact it confirms this fragmentation. Such approaches could be seen as our own theoretical symptom-formations, restrictive attempts to organize our explorations that limit our capacity to listen openly to the patient.

I would suggest a "deconstructive" rather than destructive relationship with the symptom. This begins with a commensurate validation of the suffering caused by the bulimic symptom and its organizing power, appreciating the patient's attempt to maintain the integrity of the self. As the patient discloses a world where differences have been lost, structures have collapsed, and contradictions continually arise, the therapist approaches these disclosures with two views. The creative, preserving, protective activity of the symptom-builder is validated, while the cost of the symptom to spontaneity, to experiencing the complexity of the world, and to feeling whole is explored. At the heart of this process is the empathic exploration of the patient's shame, as this feeling so often condenses experiences of neediness, hunger, the body's flaws and appetites. Shame then becomes the agent that fragments the self, while its resolution becomes the index of a new coherence of inner life. By exploring the experience of shame without recreating it, the patient begins to open new possibilities of experiencing the world. The symptom and its elaborations that have limited spontaneity and difference gradually lose their power as the patient begins to feel whole.

A vignette from the therapy of a 24-year-old student with bulimia illustrates this approach to the symptom. As she neared college graduation after a successful academic career, Gail felt trapped in a long-distance romantic relationship with Mark. She would have fantasies of his nurturing her and understanding her needs, and whenever they spent a few days together, she felt bitterly disappointed by his attempts to belittle her achievements, control her life, and his failure to understand her. She felt that he particularly valued her beauty, because it reflected well on him, like his vintage wine-cellar and his sports car. They would cycle through periods of hope, disappointment, decisions to break up, followed by a renewal of her longings for him. Her bulimic symptoms had abated through the previous year. She attributed this improvement to her increased willingness to acknowledge difficult feelings, especially aloneness. As she brought these experiences to therapy, fleshing out her self-presentation as the perfect young woman, she felt better. She struggled with her desire to be genuine in her encounters with people, but experienced setbacks that she saw as a reversion to a falseness of self when she presented herself without needs and perfectly able to emphasize with the needs of the other. We had not spoken about her symptom for quite a while.

For a month Gail became closely attached to another young woman who had a floridly symptomatic eating disorder ultimately requiring emergency hospitalization. Gail explored in displacement her shame and disgust at the symptom. For a while she did not dare to binge and purge at all, and felt enraged at her friend for having frightened her so terribly. She ended the friendship abruptly, as if she needed to purge herself of a bad part of her self.

Several months later she began to describe her shame concerning her own body. This feeling focused on her feet (she thought they were misshapen) and her breasts, which she could not allow her boyfriend or anyone else to see. She walked through a women's locker room at a health club and felt bewildered at the casual nakedness of the other women. She was so ashamed and envious that she had to run out of the room. Just before a planned vacation, she was able to tell me about an experience that occurred when she was 18, when a gynecologist told her that her breasts "sagged pathologically." He referred her for plastic surgery. Her mother said, "we must take care of this right away," but the planned surgery never occurred. During their last meeting Mark had commented about her chipped tooth as they met at the airport, and then complained about a fingernail bed that had not healed perfectly after a minor injury. He used the same words, "you should take care of that right away, have plastic surgery." She associated her sense of defectiveness, the imperfection of body parts, the experience of needing to be perfect for someone (her mother, Mark) the badness of having appetites and needs, the shame of her bulimic secret, and her shame concerning an abortion 18 months earlier. I commented on the manner in which her bulimic symptom helped her to contain and organize all of these experiences, even while it had failed to resolve her sense of shame and fragmentation. She experienced this session as a breakthrough, and left for the Caribbean.

A week later she returned. Beyond the beneficial effect vacation sometimes has on people, there was a marked transformation of her appearance. For the first time it felt to me that she was "all there." She described the vacation week as a radically different experience of herself. There had been a love affair with a man she met at the resort, moments of disclosure and intimacy with the girlfriend who accompanied her on the trip, but she also described a change in her feeling about herself. She felt lighter, even "joyful," and did not feel her usual hollowness, even when she said goodbye to her new lover. She had felt no embarrassment about being naked. She had enjoyed eating and given no thought to vomiting or feeling guilty about her meals. She had lost the need to have a binge all prepared and available any time should she crave it. She decided that she no longer needed to recycle her relationship with Mark through periods of longing and frustration, that she deserved to feel whole in any relationship she would maintain. He had consistently confirmed her defectiveness and the illegitimacy of her needs. She could now afford to give up this struggle.

Of course this moment did not signal a resolution of symptoms for this patient. It does, however, represent an experience of integration that challenges the constrained world of the bulimic symptom. Further work explored the conditions that prompted temporary reversions to that restricted world, as she moved toward the gradual elaboration of difference, complexity, and spontaneity.

This paper has explored the possibility of deconstructing the bulimic symptom: looking at a symptom in several simultaneous perspectives. The symptom is a sign, and like all signs carries a complex register of symbolic meanings. The symptom is also an act of communication, with diverse transferential addresses, whose multiplicity parallels the symbolic diversity of its meanings. In addition, the symptom is an act of mental architecture, one that both embodies and mitigates suffering. The job of the therapist who interprets the symptom, is to "deconstruct" its multiple meanings, exploring its value and its pain, to permit a more spontaneous experience of self and world that can expand the fallen-together structures of the symptomatic self.

References

Derrida, J. (1978), Freud and the scene of writing, in *Writing and Difference*, trans. A. Bass, University of Chicago Press, Chicago.

Freud, S. (1926), Inhibitions, symptoms, and anxiety, *Standard Edition*, Norton, New York, 1959.

Laplanche, J., and Pontalis, J.-B. (1973), *The Language of Psychoanalysis*, trans. D. Nicholson-Smith, Norton, New York.

Eating Disorders Unit
Massachusetts General Hospital
WACC 705
15 Parkman St.
Boston, MA 02114

INTEGRATING TREATMENTS FOR BULIMIA NERVOSA

DAVID B. HERZOG, M.D.
DEBRA L. FRANKO, PH.D.
ANDREW W. BROTMAN, M.D.

The treatment of bulimia nervosa is challenging. Bulimic patients are characteristically secretive about their symptoms and ambivalent about seeking and maintaining treatment. Moreover, bulimia nervosa is associated with significant co-morbidity and frequently coexists with other Axis I and Axis II disorders. Although bulimia nervosa, in an uncomplicated form, may respond well to cognitive, interpersonal, or psychodynamic psychotherapy or psychopharmacotherapy, this paper will focus on the refractory bulimic patient who requires an integrated multimodal treatment approach.

DSM-III-R criteria for the diagnosis of bulimia nervosa (formerly designated as bulimia in DSM-III) include at least two binge eating episodes per week for three months, a feeling of being out of control during a binge, the regular use of vomiting, laxatives, diuretics, dieting, or exercise to counteract the effect of a binge, and preoccupation with weight or body. Although bulimia nervosa can occur in individuals who are obese or underweight, most bulimics are normal weight. According to the DSM-III-R, bulimia nervosa can coexist with the diagnosis of anorexia nervosa.

The onset of this disorder frequently precedes presentation for treatment by several years. In the Eating Disorders Unit at Massachusetts General Hospital the mean duration of symptoms prior to presentation is almost six years. Typically the bulimic is ashamed of her disordered eating behaviors and has kept it a secret. Approximately 10% of the patients we see in our clinic are in ongoing psychotherapy but have not been able to inform their therapist of their disordered eating behaviors out of shame or guilt. While the bulimic is often accepting of treatment initially, she may have a low

David B. Herzog is an Associate Professor of Psychiatry; Debra L. Franko is an Instructor in Psychiatry (Psychology); Andrew W. Brotman is an Assistant Professor of Psychiatry, all at Harvard Medical School.

tolerance for frustration and quickly terminate treatment when it does not provide immediate symptomatic relief.

A thorough psychiatric evaluation is essential to determining the best method of treatment for an individual bulimic patient. She may have concomitant major affective disorder, anxiety disorder, substance-use disorder, kleptomania, or personality disorder. In our clinical population, nearly a quarter of the patients have made a major suicide attempt.

Often, however, the patients we see have several coexisting diagnoses or are persistently symptomatic despite years of intensive psychodynamic psychotherapy. These patients require an integrated multimodal treatment approach grounded in a therapeutic relationship over an extended period of time. Such an approach uses cognitive-behavioral and/or biologic treatments to provide both structure and symptom reduction that in turn support the ongoing psychotherapy.

Why would we recommend an integrated treatment program for bulimia nervosa? This eating disorder is an admixture of thoughts, behaviors, and affects. There are behavioral components (binge eating, vomiting, fasting), cognitive aberrations (irrational beliefs concerning weight, food, and body image), and psychodynamic underpinnings (deficits at various developmental levels). As well, this disorder often results in serious medical complications as a consequence of these behaviors. Finally, because it is a disorder of eating, nutritional concerns are present. Thus, the multidimensional nature of the disorder itself demonstrates the need for an integrative approach in psychotherapy.

Although we recognize other forms of treatment as potentially useful (e.g., behavior therapy, self-help groups) we will focus on three treatment modalities: psychodynamic, cognitive-behavioral, and pharmocologic. The frequency with which psychodynamic psychotherapy is prescribed punctuates the importance of its discussion. Cognitive-behavioral and pharmacologic therapies have received substantial empirical support for their effectiveness, at least in the short term (Garfinkel and Garner, 1987; Wilson et al., 1986). A short description of these three modalities in the treatment of bulimia nervosa will serve as the background for our discussion of an integrated treatment approach.

The focus of psychodynamically oriented therapy for bulimia nervosa has evolved from psychosexual formulations to object relations and disturbances of self and identity. (Swift and Letven, 1984). Current psychodynamic understanding and treatment of bulimia nervosa examine the symptomatology in tension regulation. Treatment issues include: the id anxiety states and negative emotion; recollections of giving environment particularly as it attended to affective homeostasis, and soothing; and the use self-objects. Therapy involves the identification of temperment variables in the patient and early caregivers as well as of external stressors that may have influenced the balance and comfort attainable in the patient's early years. Other frequent themes include: the patient's and family's use of food and orality in achieving homeostasis and palliating affect, the family's limits on appetites of all kinds, and the definitions of fullness and satiety in eating and emotion. Dependency and separation-individualization are common developmental conflicts. Many patients have idealized their families and adopted a false self defined by parents' needs and expectations rather than on their own personas. Early traumatic experiences are often present yet unexpressed (loss, abuse, failure), the pain never explored and affective homeostasis never achieved. Numbness pervades in order to manage anxiety, and eating becomes disordered. Determining the underlying meaning of the bulimic symptoms and the functions they serve for the patient are primary goals of psychodynamic therapy. In time, the patient learns appropriate ways to identify, express, and regulate affect and begins to use the therapist, then significant others, as self-objects.

Studies on cognitive-behavioral treatment for bulimia first appeared in 1981 with Fairburn's paper documenting the effectiveness of this approach (Fairburn, 1981). Cognitive-behavioral treatment focuses on the use of several techniques to change both the bulimic behaviors and the dysfunctional attitudes that accompany them. These techniques include self-monitoring, meal planning, attitudinal restructuring, and discussion of the association between mood states and binging. The goals of this form of treatment are symptom control and alteration of the cognitive distortions concerning food, weight, and body shape (Garner et al., 1987).

Pharmacological treatments have received increasing attention after several published studies reported the effectiveness of antidepressant medications in the short treatment of bulimia (Garfinkel and Garner, 1987; Hughes et al., 1986). The goal of introducing medication into the treatment is the reduction of symptom(s) of bulimia and/or depression. It is unclear whether these drugs have a pecific antibinge action or work through the treatment of the depressive symptomatology.

Despite the enthusiasm for the use of antidepressants in the treatment of bulimia nervosa, the only published long-term study suggests that the antibulimic effect of antidepressants may not persist over time. Therefore, patients may require multiple successive antidepressant trials in order to maintain or improve response (Pope et al., 1985). Furthermore, follow-up reports suggest that bulimics may be particularly susceptible to the side effects of medications, and often choose to go off these medications even when they are effective. Bulimic patients, in addition, are often resistant to accepting medication. They express concerns that they may get hooked on the drug, that drugs are an artificial way of treating the problem, that they may get fat, or that taking medication means that they are extremely disturbed. We have found that excessive weight gain and carbohydrate cravings are not common side effects among bulimics treated with antidepressants. We believe that antidepressants plus psychotherapy are more effective than either modality alone in most complex cases. We do not recommend psychotropic medication as the sole intervention.

Psychodynamic psychotherapy, cognitive-behavioral therapy and pharmacotherapy have the explicit goal of symptom relief. However, their implicit goals are different: exploration and understanding of early relationships and the meaning of symptoms, behavioral and cognitive change, and normalization of biologic functions respectively. How to integrate such apparently disparate treatments may be difficult to perceive.

Several approaches to integrating the treatments of bulimia nervosa are possible. Symptoms can be addressed early in treatment using cognitive-behavioral therapy. Once some symptom control is achieved, the focus can be shifted to underlying psychodynamic issues. Alternatively, cognitive-behavioral, psychodynamic, and psychopharmacological techniques can be used simultaneously over the course of treatment. Finally, an integrated perspective can be achieved by using the therapeutic relationship as the unifying context in which all activity is understood and examined.

The first task for the therapist is to determine what forms of treatment are appropriate at the outset and how integration will proceed. Many prescriptions are possible and treatment needs change over time. The therapist must be flexible enough to "tailor" the treatment for each patient in content as well as timing. For example, the bulimic patient may have stopped binging and purging altogether, yet may continue to have a severely distorted image of her body size and shape. Therapy may shift from a discussion of symptoms to an active exploration of her feelings about herself, the early messages she received from significant others regarding her body, and an examination of her dysfunctional attitudes and beliefs.

We present one therapeutic technique and several case examples to illustrate the concept of integration and to offer an approach for the treatment of the refractory bulimic patient.

Food diaries are a powerful behavioral tool. Patients are asked to record the events, thoughts, and feelings that occur before and after an episode of binging and purging. Notably, of the eight cognitive-behavioral groups one of us has conducted (D.F.), the lowest dropout rate occurred in the group in which food diaries were commented on and returned to the patients each week. Food diaries can also be useful from a psychodynamic perspective. They serve as transitional objects by offering the patient some control when the therapist is not available. Diaries also provide material for elaboration of thoughts and feelings that precede or accompany bulimic behaviors, setting the stage for further exploration of psychodynamic issues. Finally, they can be used to address the issue of control by providing patients with concrete evidence that the urge to binge is not an isolated phenomenon but can be connected with emotions and thoughts.

Case Example 1

A 25-year-old single white female graduate student sought cognitive-behavioral treatment for bulimia nervosa of eight years duration. She was binging approximately five times per day, and had recently terminated psychodynamic psychotherapy with her therapist of seven years because of persistent bulimic symptoms and a disagreement over whether to utilize alternative treatment approaches. Behavioral strategies, including use of behavioral logs, meal planning, short-term goal contracts, lists of alternative activities, time delay techniques, and time structuring planning resulted in a 50% diminution of bulimic symptoms within four weeks. However, the patient remained symptomatic and continued to binge twice a day. Evaluation also demonstrated that she was depressed, although she fell short of meeting full criteria for major depressive disorder. Antidepressant medication was added to cognitive-behavioral treatment, and the patient was titrated up to a dose of 200 mg of desipramine per day over the next three weeks. After approximately six weeks on a therapeutic dose, her bulimic symptomatology continued to improve. Binge-purge episodes were reduced to approximately twice per week. Her depressive and anxious symptoms also improved. At this stage of treatment, the predominant mode of therapy switched back to a psychodynamic orientation, concentrating on her self-esteem, interpersonal relations, and family history. Cognitive-behavioral techniques continued to be used as needed. After several months of treatment, the patient was binging and purging no more than once per week. Medication was tapered on two occasions over the next year, with a resultant increase in depressive symptoms and an increase in bulimic symptomatology to approximately three of four times per week. She continues on a maintenance dose of desipramine 150 mg per day, receiving cognitive behavioral techniques as needed, while being engaged in predominantly psychodynamic psychotherapy.

This case demonstrates several points. First of all, although psychodynamic psychotherapy was definitely useful in a severely symptomatic individual for the seven years prior to coming into an alternative treatment, the bulimic sypmtoms needed to be addressed directly. Adherence to a strict psychodynamic theoretical orientation in the midst of severe symptomatology was not useful, leading to the end of a long-term therapeutic relationship. Second, this case demonstrates that the integration of multiple therapies can result in a rather rapid and significant reduction in symptomatology even in the case of a chronic bulimic with both an affective and a personality disorder who has made only modest changes despite long-term psychodynamic psychotherapy. This reduction may in turn enhance the effectiveness of psychodynamic psychotherapy.

Case Example 2

A 31-year-old married mother of two presented for treatment. She had a two-year history of bulimia nervosa involving approximately 14 binge-purge episodes per week. In addition, she complained of marital difficulty, periodic suicidal ideation, and obsessive-compulsive symptoms characterized by the belief that she was dirty and needed constantly to wash. Her husband refused to come in for treatment, so the patient was started in individual psychodynamically oriented psychotherapy. When her symptoms persisted for several months, she also entered a long-term psychodynamic psychotherapy group for bulimics. Her bulimia decreased by about 50%, but she continued to have periodic suicidal depression and obsessive-compulsive symptoms. At this point, she underwent pharmacologic consultation and was placed on the monoamine oxidase inhibitor, phenelzine, at therapeutic doses. With these three approaches she continued to improve and her bulimia was in full remission within several months. She terminated the group and continued in individual psychotherapy with medication. The psychotherapy focused on her low self-esteem and her obsessions. After eight months, medication was tapered. At four year follow-up she has had no recurrence of either bulimia or obsessive-compulsive symptoms and has been off medication for seven months. She continues in psychotherapy once monthly.

This situation is another in which a patient had multiple diagnoses including bulimia nervosa, obsessive-compulsive disorder, major depression, and a mixed personality disorder. In this case cognitive behavioral approaches were only minimally used in a group setting. The patient's personality problems and bulimia improved with individual and group therapy. However, the addition of a monoamine oxidase inhibitor afforded her increased control and ultimately total remission of her bulimia with some relief from her obsessions and compulsions. She made substantial progress in ongoing psychotherapy and, when the medication was discontinued, she remained symptom free. Dynamic psychotherapy was the predominant mode of treatment, leading to the elimination of depressive episodes with suicidal ideation. Pharmacotherapy was helpful as well in providing some control over her acute symptomatology. This control enabled her to do the interpretive work that could create structural intrapsychic change. This change, in turn, would facilitate more effective tension regulation and improved self-esteem.

Case Example 3

A 33-year-old married woman requested behavior therapy for bulimic symptoms that had persisted over ten years. Cognitive-behavioral therapy was offered and the patient completed food diaries, planned regular meals, and began to examine her distortions about her body size and weight. She stopped binging after several weeks, but continued to feel the urge to vomit, even after a small meal. A suggestion to delay the vomiting by increasing intervals of time (five minutes one day, then ten minutes, etc.) created a great deal of anxiety in the patient. The thoughts and feelings she experienced while attempting to carry out this intervention led to a greater understanding of her symptoms. In describing her experience, she became aware that after eating that she would "explode and disintegrate," as if the food inside her would make her burst. She then recalled that her mother's constant demands during her childhood often made her so angry she feared losing control and exploding in rage. She was able to observe that the vomiting was a way of relieving this anxiety by eliminating the feeling of fullness that precipitated it. Within several months of combined psychodynamic exploration and cognitive-behavioral techniques, her binging and purging decreased significantly.

This case illustrates the point that it is important to respond to a request from the patient. This patient asked for behavior therapy; the therapist should be flexible enough to answer that request even though it may be clear that psychodynamic issues are at the core of the symptomatology. This patient was not ready to discuss the influence of her mother during the initial stages of treatment; however, by meeting her request for a behavioral intervention, such issues eventually surfaced. Moreover, active behavioral techniques, specifically directives, may influence the transference. In this case, since the patient perceived her mother as demanding and intrusive, the therapist's request for behavioral logs may have intensified the transference. Although the behavioral interventions may have led to symptom remission, it is also possible that the interpretation and clarification of the transference contributed to the favorable outcome.

In patients whose severe bulimia is accompanied by a personality disorder, psychodynamic psychotherapy is conducted on a relatively long-term basis. Cognitive behavioral techniques and pharmacotherapy are used as needed. When major affective disorder is chronic or recurrent, maintenance medication should be considered. In most cases cognitive behavioral techniques are strategically used to manage bulimic symptoms that break through under certain stressors. In our view these three approaches are compatible, particularly for the individual with significant co-morbidity.

The greatest impediment to integration occurs when the theoretical orientation of primary therapists causes them to reject or overlook other treatment modalities. Many psychiatrists are not familiar with all three approaches, and nonphysicians clearly require consultants when pharmacotherapy is employed. Therefore, if more than one person is providing treatment, it is essential that they work with mutual respect and tolerance toward the common goals of symptom relief and resolution for the patient. For example, rigid adherence to the psychodynamic or cognitive-behavioral orientation may cause a practitioner to overlook or undercut pharmacological approaches. The patient may be given the impression that use of medication is not an option or represents failure. Conversely, overreliance on psychopharmacologic views may ignore important dynamic issues necessary to the treatment.

Our view is that bulimia nervosa is often a complicated disorder and, when complicated, requires more than one treatment modality. The multiple modalities can be integrated only if all practioners understand their roles and respect different modes of intervention. Psychotherapy is the primary treatment matrix through which all other modalities are introduced and monitored. Pharmacotherapy is recommended for the bulimic who has concomitant major depressive disorder, manic depressive illness, substantial depressive or anxiety symptomatology, obsessive-compulsive symptomatology, or who has been resistent to usual psychotherapeutic interventions and continues to have distressing bulimic symptomatology. Cognitive-behavioral treatment techniques often are useful to establish a sense of control and to monitor symptoms both early in treatment and during relapses.

Multimodal management of complicated cases of bulimia nervosa is a challenge. Yet, this method offers the clinician a problem-oriented sequential approach to otherwise elusive cases. The many pieces to the puzzle of this disorder can be as overwhelming and elusive to the clinician as they are to the patient. Where does one begin? How does one approach these complex cases? The interweaving of sometimes disparate theories and therapies by the clinician provides not only the real help needed by the patient but symbolic modeling of what the patient herself must do internally. It is through experiencing the successful integration of effective treatments that the patient begins to feel "adequate caregiving" for her disorder. Thus, she gains an emergent sense of emotional homeostasis about her symptoms and their causes. As the patient subsequently begins her own psychic reintegration of the pieces of her disorder, she can approach a sense of healing, balance, and emotional integrity within herself. It is this outcome that makes the integration of treatments for complex bulimia nervosa most worthwhile.

References

Fairburn, C. G. (1981), A cognitive behavioral approach to the management of bulimia, *Psychol. Med., 11*, 707–711.

Garner, D. M., Fairburn, C. G., and Davids, R. (1987), Cognitive-behavioral treatment of bulimia nervosa: A critical appraisal, *Behav. Modi., 11*, 398–431.

Garfinkel, P. E., Garner, D. M. (1987), *The Role of Drug Treatment for Disorders*, Brunner/Mazel, New York.

Herzog, D. B., Hamburg, P., and Brotman, A. W. (1987), Commentary: Psychotherapy and eating disorders: An affirmative view, *Int. J. Eating Disorders, 6*, 545–550.

Hughes, P. L., Wells, L. A., and Cunningham, C. J. (1986), Treating bulimia with desipramine: A double-blind, placebo-controlled study, *Arch. Gen. Psychiatry, 43*, 182–186.

Pope, H. G., Hudson, J. I., and Jonas, J. M. (1985), Antidepressant treatment of bulimia: A two-year follow-up study, *J. Clini. Psychopharma., 5*, 320–327.

Swift, W. J., and Letvin, R. (1984), Bulimia and the basic fault: A psychoanalytic interpretation of the binging-vomiting syndrome, *J. Am. Acad. Child Psychiatry, 23*, 489–497.

Wilson, G. T., Rossiter, E., Kleifield, E., and Lindholm, L. (1986), Cognitive-behavioral treatment of bulimia nervosa: A controlled evaluation. *Behav. Res. Ther., 24*, 277–288.

Eating Disorders Unit
Massachusetts General Hospital, WACC 625
15 Parkman Street
Boston, MA 02114

OBESITY: A PSYCHOANALYTIC CHALLENGE

MYRON L. GLUCKSMAN, M.D.

The purpose of this paper is to examine obesity from a psychoanalytic perspective in the context of current theoretical, clinical, and biological knowledge. Obesity is usually defined in terms of body weight and includes those individuals who are 20% or more above their optimal weight, or who have 20% or more of their body weight composed of adipose tissue. Categories of obesity are based on the age of onset, types of abnormal eating patterns, and the degree of body-image disturbance. From a psychiatric standpoint, obesity is neither psychopathologically nor developmentally a uniform syndrome. Yet, the literature seems to suggest a common psychodynamic thread, especially in connection with "developmental" or "childhood onset" obesity. Those psychoanalysts who initially explored the psychogenesis of obesity linked it to disturbances in the oral phase of development (Alexander, 1934; Bychowski, 1950; Hamburger, 1951; Rascovsky et al., 1950). Freud's (1905) concept of an oral erotogenic zone promoting sexual pleasure independent of nutritional requirements was the foundation of this hypothesis. The latter held that excesses or deficiencies of oral stimulation during infancy led to partial or total "fixations" at the oral stage of development. These "fixations" were the result of either too much or too little pleasurable gratification during the oral phase. Therefore, the infant who failed to obtain an appropriate amount of oral gratification might regress to an oral level of behavior under future stressful circumstances. Examples of oral behavior include overeating, thumbsucking, smoking, drinking, and other types of orally devouring activities. Over time, the concept of oral gratification was broadened to include the infant's total kinesthetic, visual, auditory, and affective experience with the mother during the earliest stage of development. Since feeding is so central an activity during infancy, every component of the mother–child relationship can become associated with food and eating. Significant impairment of mother–child interac-

---

Myron L. Glucksman is a Clinical Professor, Department of Psychiatry, New York Medical College and an Associate Clinical Professor, Department of Psychiatry, Yale University School of Medicine.

tion, including the feeding process, can possibly lead to oral "fixation." This means that future emotional distress might result in excessive eating or other oral activities in an attempt to recreate optimal maternal care and comforting.

Levy (1934) suggested that "affect hunger" was the cause of eating disorders in adulthood. He defined "affect hunger" as the "emotional hunger for maternal love and the other feelings of being cared for in the mother–child relationship." According to Levy, obese individuals project "affect hunger" onto food as the tangible form of the mother, thereby mothering themselves in order to feel secure and to fill up their "structural emptiness." Levy's "affect hunger" appears to be closely related to Winnicott's (1953) concept of the transitional object as a "soother" or "sedative" when the mother is absent. For the obese individual, food may act as a transitional object for the purpose of defending against feelings originally connected with separation from the mother (e.g., anxiety, loneliness). Winnicott (1971) observed that feeding progresses from an initial stage of undifferentiation where the baby and breast are not perceived as separate, to a later awareness of feeding from an "other than me" source. A proper feeding experience with a "good-enough mother" promotes the development of the infant's capacity for healthy object differentiation and the ability to love. According to Winnicott (1965) and others (Kohut, 1971; Mahler et al., 1975; Spitz, 1965), satisfactory feeding experiences are a basic requirement toward the development of normal object relations and the evolution of a cohesive, stable sense of self. Anna Freud (1972) believed that food and mother became consciously separated in children by the age of two, although the unconscious equation remains intact. Bruch (1957) observed that the mothers of obese children interfere with normal developmental differentiation between self and object. According to her, the obesegenic mother maintains an overprotective, dependency-inducing attitude toward her child as if it were a prized, inanimate possession. She offers food overabundantly and inappropriately for nonnutritional reasons; for example, as a substitute for other needs of the child that she cannot satisfy or for her own dependency needs. Becuase of this excessive and inappropriate feeding, obese children suffer from perceptual and conceptual disturbances. Specifically, they are unable to distinguish between hunger, satiation, and other internal somatic sensations, including feelings. Bruch is in agreement with other investigators who emphasize the importance of maternal "attunement" for the infant's healthy development (Kohut, 1971, 1977; Modell, 1976; Ornstein, 1981; Tolpin, 1971). This means that the mother must differentiate the child's needs from her own in the setting of an adequate "holding environment," an atmosphere in which the mother is sensitive as well as responsive to the infant's needs, thereby promoting an internalization of the maternal soothing function. Thus, the child's capacity for self-soothing is a consequence of empathic maternal responses that create a healthy matrix of self-objects. This process enables the child to develop self-cohesion, object constancy, and the ability to tolerate separation from the mother. Goodsitt (1983) concludes that obese individuals have experienced failures in empathic mirroring leading to an inability to self-soothe when feeling anxious, depressed, or lonely. Their addictive craving for food results in temporary self-soothing, but it fails to build psychological structure or self-cohesion. According to this theory, obese persons have a limited capacity for self-soothing and overeat in order to reproduce a sensorimotor representation of the mother and her soothing activities, which have not been properly internalized.

There are two major clinical disturbances characteristic of obese individuals: (1) abnormal eating patterns, and (2) body-image pathology. Hyperphagia without the ordinary sensation of hunger is the most salient feature of their deviant eating behavior. Clinical and experimental evidence suggests that they are unable to identify the physical sensations of hunger and satiety correctly (Bruch, 1961; Stunkard and Koch, 1964). However, they compulsively overeat in association with a variety of emotional states, and in connection with a multiplicity of psychodynamic issues. Kaplan and Kaplan (1957) observed 27 affective and psychodynamic factors significantly correlated with overeating. These included anxiety, anger, guilt, depression, self-punishment, self-reward, insecurity, defiance, feeling unloved, seeking attention, avoiding competition, and the like. They point out that almost any unresolved psychodynamic conflict arising at each stage of psychosexual development can be linked to overeating. In my clinical investigations I have been impressed with the close relationship between hyperphagia and various dysphoric states associated with numerous psychodynamic issues that are the sequelae of disturbances at the oral and post-oral stages of development (Glucksman, 1968, 1972; Glucksman et al., 1978). Some investigators emphasize that overeating is primarily a means of coping with emotional distress and minimize the specific psychodynamics involved. Slochower (1983) describes several studies that suggest that obese subjects overeat in response to a variety of "uncontrollable emotional states." They are unable to cope with painful emotions because they are unable to "label them" (similar to Bruch's observations), leading to a sense of helplessness rather than mastery. Others (Castelnuovo-Tedesco and Reiser, 1988) contend that obesity and compulsive eating constitute an addictive or impulse disorder. They view overeating as a self-soothing activity that provides "substitute gratification." The latter is an attempt to replace lost or disappointing love objects, and to recreate a preverbal attachment to the mother. Addictive eating behavior is a way of coping with dysphoria, particularly empty, lonely, yearning feelings. These observations are similar to Khantzian's (1985) studies of drug-dependent individuals. He maintains that narcotic addicts choose opiates because they calm their aggressive, violent feelings, while cocaine addicts use cocaine because it relieves feelings of depression, boredom, and emptiness. Therefore compulsive eating, similar to drug addiction, can be viewed as a form of self-medication in order to allay painful emotions. Raynes (1987) observed that overweight women manifest less well-developed internal representations of their mothers than their fathers on psychological test assessment. She hypothesizes that they overeat in response to specific distressing emotions (e.g., anxiety, loneliness) in order to compensate for inadequately internalized maternal functions, including self-soothing and "anxiety management." In general, there is substantial clinical as well as experimental evidence that overeating is a maladaptive attempt to reduce painful affects and to restore a sense of well-being by using food as a symbolic representation of maternal soothing functions.

Body image, an important component of self-image, refers to the mental representation of one's body along with the attitudes, feelings, fantasies, and conflicts associated with it. Clinically, body-image disturbances in obese patients fall into two categories: (1) Primary body-image disturbances, and (2) body-image abnormalities secondary to being obese. Primary body-image disturbances are intimately connected to problems of self-representation. For example, a large body size (fatness) can be a physical manifestation of an inner sense of worthlessness, unloveability, and inferiority. Patients who suffer from childhood-onset obesity are more likely to have primary body-image disturbances because of developmental difficulties leading to pathology of the self. Internal feelings of emptiness, vulnerability, and self-fragmentation may be defended against by perceiving oneself to be huge and impenetrable. Bruch (1957) believes that obese children need to experience themselves as big and powerful because they are compensating for the unfulfilled desires or wishes of their parents. A consistent finding in obese patients is that they have considerable difficulty in estimating their body size (Glucksman and Hirsch, 1969). They frequently overestimate their body size and believe that they are still fat even after losing a significant amount of weight. This is particularly true for patients with childhood-onset obesity, since body-size representation becomes relatively fixed during adolescence.

Secondary body-image disturbances are a consequence of being obese in a society that places a high value on thinness. Obese individuals are subject to a constant barrage from the media, advertising, and fashion that connects thinness with desirability and acceptance, while overweight is linked to unacceptability and rejection. Thus, almost all obese individuals view their bodies with some degree of self-loathing and self-derogation. These feelings are often projected onto others who are obese. Body size may also be employed defensively in a number of ways; for example, some obese patients utilize their body size to intimidate and control others, or symbolically to protect themselves from interpersonal injury (physical or psychological) Obesity may also be used as a rationalization for failure at one's career or in social and sexual relationships.

An informative study conducted under the auspices of the American Academy of Psychoanalysis examined the outcome of psychoanalytic treatment for obesity (Rand and Stunkard, 1977, 1978, 1983). It is one of the few studies carried out to date that has included control and experimental populations in order to investigate the efficacy of psychoanalytic treatment. The study consisted of 147 patients: 64 obese women, 20 obese men (experimental group), as well as 46 normal-weight women and 17 normal-weight men (control group). At the end of 4 years, 66% of the obese patients lost more than 20 pounds, and 25% lost more than 40 pounds. These results compare quite favorably with other forms of treatment for obesity (e.g., behavioral, peer support). The study clearly established that there are specific psychodynamic constellations associated with weight gain, weight loss, and deviant eating patterns for obese patients. There was also a significant reduction in the intensity of body-image disparagement that seemed to be more the result of therapy than of weight loss.

Further analysis of the data in this study revealed that the psychodynamic factors could be classified under several distinct categories: (1) mood or affect, (2) self- and body image, (3) psycho-dynamic issues related to deprivation and gratification, (4) psycho-dynamic issues involved with aggression or competition, and (5) sexual conflicts (Glucksman et al., 1978). Specific psychodynamic conflicts in each of these categories were associated with weight gain, weight loss, and abnormal eating patterns with significantly greater frequency for the obese than for the normal-weight patients. Unresolved psychodynamic conflicts ("negative" psychodynamics) were more frequently observed with overeating and weight gain, while psychodynamic conflicts that had been resolved ("positive" psychodynamics) were more frequently connected with normal eating behavior and weight loss. For example, weight gain was associated with poor self-esteem and feelings of inadequacy, while weight loss was correlated with increased self-esteem and feelings of competence. The psychodynamic constellation observed with greatest frequency in the obese population involved issues of deprivation and gratification. As an example, during periods of weight gain patients often expressed feelings of being unloved and disappointed in their interpersonal relationships. However, during periods of weight loss they reported greater satisfaction in their relationships. In general, treatment enabled the obese patients to tolerate painful emotions better, particularly those connected with abandonment and separation (e.g., sadness, loneliness). They were also able to change their perception of self- and body image in the direction of greater self-esteem and less derogation of their body size.

I have treated one of the patients who participated in the Academy Study for the past 14 years. This has afforded me the opportunity to explore in much greater depth the various psychodynamics connected with obesity than the questionnaire methodology of the study permitted. In presenting this patient, I shall focus on the psychodynamics associated with compulsive eating, weight fluctuations, self-representation and body image. I shall also attempt to integrate these psychodynamic factors with current genetic, metabolic, morphologic, and neurochemical data.

CASE PRESENTATION

The patient is a 47-year-old married professional woman who entered treatment because of obesity, dissatisfaction with her job, marital difficulties, poor self-esteem, and a pervasive sense of unhappiness. She weighed 226 pounds at the outset of therapy. Her obesity began in mid-adolescence and has continued throughout adulthood. Despite numerous diets, Weight Watchers, and appetite suppressants she was unable to lose any significant amounts of weight prior to treatment. She has three children, two sons and one daughter. Her marriage has been stable, although she has never felt fully satisfied with her husband intellectually, emotionally, or sexually. Her parents are living, but she has never felt a close bond to them, particularly to her mother. Her father became obese as an adult, but her mother and an older sister have always been thin or normal-weight. I have divided her treatment into three phases, based on weight changes and psychodynamic issues.

Phase 1

During the initial phase of treatment she quickly formed a good working alliance and a positive transference. She felt that I was empathic and supportive, in contrast to her husband whom she portrayed as insensitive, superficial, and financially irresponsible. Their sexual relationship was sporadic and generally unsatisfying for her. Her eating pattern was characterized by binging and between-meal-eating, usually in connection with unpleasant feelings. However, she sometimes found herself overeating when feeling neutral or even in a pleasant mood. It became apparent that she viewed herself in terms of either a thin self or a fat self. She was disgusted by her fat self and loathed her appearance. As a fat person she felt unloveable, inadequate, and sexually repulsive. On the other hand, she fantasized her thin self to be attractive, worthwhile, and sexually desirable. Yet, her actual weight precluded sexual flirtations as well as the possibility of being found attractive by men. Nevertheless, within the first year of treatment she revealed her fantasy of seducing me when she reached 150 pounds. This fantasy partly fueled a self-imposed dieting regimen during which she lost 60 pounds over the first two years of therapy. Additional details of her family history emerged over this period. She was bottle-fed as an infant and was normal-weight throughout childhood. Food was not used by her parents as a reward for accomplishments or good behavior, but she was always encouraged to "clean her plate." For as long as she could remember, her mother seemed emotionally distant, critical, and uninterested in how she felt. She could not recall her mother ever telling her she loved her. Her father was more supportive, but her mother always seemed to interfere with her attempts to be close to him. He displayed open affection for her only when he was intoxicated. She began to gain excessive weight at age 15 when the family moved to a different town where she felt lonely and socially excluded by her classmates at a new school.

At the end of 2 years of treatment she weighed 165 pounds. She decided to terminate therapy because she felt less depressed and was close to her desired weight. At the same time, she was annoyed with me for taking a "neutral" attitude in regard to her weight loss and proposed termination. The following dream occurred in this context: "I was watching my EKG—my heart slowed and I asked for a pacemaker. I couldn't get one and my heart stopped. I died."

The dream conveyed her underlying feelings about termination: she felt that she would emotionally "die" without my availability to help her understand and resolve her problems. When I did not interfere with her plans to terminate, she believed that I truly did not care about her and became enraged at me. Following our exploration of this dream she decided to continue treatment.

Phase 2

This phase of treatment was characterized by an intensely ambivalent transference and a prolonged struggle to come to terms with the thin and fat components of her self-representation. She was alternately angry at me for failing to help her change her negative self-image, yet grateful for my acceptance of her undesirable qualities. Her fat self overshadowed her thin self, and she continually berated herself for being stupid, lazy, incompetent, and unattractive. As her fortieth birthday approached she entertained fantasies of becoming pregnant in order to prove her youthfulness and fertility. While having intercourse with her husband she fantasized that I was impregnating her. It became clear that this was a way of incorporating me, enabling her to permanently continue her attachment to me. The baby, a displacement of myself, would provide her with my love and attention long after she terminated treatment. In addition, she could give the baby the kind of emotional closeness and loving that her mother failed to give her. Predictably, she became pregnant but had an abortion once she understood her unconscious needs for the baby, as well as the difficulties it would present at her stage of life. However, following the abortion, she became depressed and guilt-ridden. A lengthy period of grieving ensued, accompanied by a considerable increase in weight.

Oedipal themes were introduced by a dream in which she "witnessed something [she] shouldn't have." She recalled having slept in the same bedroom as her parents until age 6. Her father's genitalia were a source of curiosity and excitement for her. Memories emerged of feeling sexually aroused while sitting on his lap, hugging, and kissing him. Further dreams and fantasies centered around competitive feelings toward other women, her expectation of their retaliatory behavior, and her defenses against them. These included an avoidance of self-assertion or confrontation with female authorities and peers at work. Moreover, her obesity was a signal to other women that she posed no threat to them since their was little likelihood that men would find her attractive. Her first sexual relationship was with an older man with whom she worked at a summer job. She confided in her sister who, in turn, told her mother. A swift reproach by her mother still rings in her ears: "How could you!" She became terrified of her mother's anger in connection with any future sexual relationships.

Further exploration elicited feelings of terror and powerlessness in regard to her mother when she was a young child. According to the patient, her mother "ruled like a queen and no one was allowed to argue or disagree with her unless you were prepared to face her wrath." When the family moved and she transferred to a new school at the age of 15 she was socially rejected by her peers. Without her mother's support or understanding, she felt humiliated, sad, and alone. Eating became a source of comfort, and she began to gain weight.

As treatment progressed, dream content and fantasy material increasingly reflected pre-oedipal themes. The following dream was representative:

> I went into my childhood bedroom and saw my mother in bed. I felt sexually aroused, but she told me to take a bath before I got in bed with her. When I returned my husband was in bed instead of my mother. I was disappointed, yet went ahead and made love with him. I didn't feel anything.

She recalled how much she wanted to be loved and praised by her mother as a child, but instead was met with indifference and "perfunctory" kisses. She described having homosexual fantasies in which other women gave her the warmth, affection, and understanding she yearned for. These fantasies expressed her wish to be loved as well as understood by her mother, and functioned as a defense against heterosexual fantasies that evoked oedipally related anxiety. Sexual intercourse with her husband was not totally satisfying because it was far more important to be held and caressed. She described a recurrent fantasy of lying in a hospital bed gravely ill, being comforted, and taken care of by me. In subsequent dreams and fantasies I played dual roles: a forbidden, incestuous love object and a comforting maternal figure. Her self-image and sexual fantasies oscillated between viewing herself as thin, successful, and sexually attractive, or as obese, worthless, and sexually repulsive. As a thin person she would seduce me, divorce her husband, and live with me. The anxiety associated with this fantasy was defended against by another fantasy where she saw herself as obese, lesbian, and in a comforting, nurturing relationship with another woman.

During this phase of therapy her weight fluctuated between 190 and 210 pounds. She resented me for not taking a more active role in supervising her attempts to diet. I responded by saying that although I understood her torment over her weight, I did not wish to become either an advocate or an opponent of any part of herself. She interpreted my response as evidence of my indifference to her weight problem, and maintained that I secretly loathed her appearance. I suggested that I reminded her of her mother who, at best, behaved indifferently toward her, and at worst, treated her with disgust. She replied: "If I were thin my mother (you) would love me . . . it's impossible to get my mother's (your) love as I am . . . why can't she (you) appreciate and love me as I am?" Toward the end of this phase of treatment she attended a weight loss spa on two occasions and cumulatively lost 25 pounds. She felt pleased with her appearance and once again entertained the possibility of termination. A pivotal dream occurred at this time:

> My cat was drinking from the toilet and fell in. I got so angry that I flushed the toilet in order to clean him. He jumped out — I realized that I could have killed him. I felt guilty and became aware of how much I loved him.

She identified the cat with herself, and flushing the toilet was her wish to terminate therapy. However, she knew she couldn't terminate because she still required my help. I was apparently allowing her to terminate — "to drown" — and I seemed unconcerned. My alleged attitude enraged her and she wanted to kill me (in this case, I was the cat), yet was compelled to save both of us by having the cat jump out. She stated: "I need to come here — I need your love but that's forbidden so I have to get rid of it, flush it (you) down the toilet . . . but I want to be close to you, to have your love, respect and understanding." Further associations concerned binging, vomiting, and flushing it down the toilet. Eating voraciously (binging) was a symbolic way of incorporating me as well as her mother, and gaining our love. However, my love was forbidden and dangerous because it evoked anxiety connected with oedipal wishes. By flushing the toilet she simultaneously rid herself of the object of her incestuous impulses (myself) as well as her potentially punishing mother. In addition to its oedipal and preoedipal components, the dream portrayed various aspects of herself. The cat represented parts of herself she wished to destroy (fatness, sexual unattractiveness, social and professional inadequacy) and parts of herself she hoped to promote (normal weight, sexual attractiveness, professional competence, social acceptance). The resolution of the "cat dream" in favor of survival and continued self-growth reflected a significant turning point in her therapy.

Phase 3

This phase was characterized by greater self-acceptance, and a more realistic perception of her parents as well as of myself. Her self-esteem was enhanced when she was offered a position at work that she had fantasized about for several years. The fact that her professional ability was publicly recognized significantly buoyed her self-confidence. We continued to explore the connections between her feelings, different aspects of herself, and her compulsive eating. Food enabled her to fill the emotional emptiness she felt in her relationship with her parents and her husband. Her sessions with me helped to fill the void, but it became apparent that I had become a transitional object or "food" that she incorporated in order to feel emotionally understood and accepted. Subsequent dream and fantasy material centered around being treated and valued by me as my equal. In one dream, I came to visit her and was impressed by her books as well as other objects in her house. She took great pleasure in my appreciation of her intellect and her good taste in art. An important issue in the dream was that she appeared as her obese self and yet I still admired her: "I looked the way I am and you still liked me — it was enough for you to want to stay with me." In the following months she was gradually able to distinguish and separate her bodily self from other parts of her self-representation. During this process she realized the extent to which her obese, physical self was the externalized, reified manifestation of her internal, unacceptable qualities. Her actual weight, though still an important issue for her, received less of our attention. Her "good" and "bad" qualities, similar to her "thin" and "fat" selves, became more integrated into a cohesive, acceptable self. She gradually accepted her parents' limitations, and relinquished the fantasy of her mother giving her the overt, unqualified love and approval she longed for. Recently, her father (while sober) told her that he loved her, and acknowledged that her mother had "problems" showing affection. Her father's demonstration of his love for her as well as his validation of her mother's limitations, helped her to consolidate a sense of being worthwhile and loveable. At this point in treatment she weighed 250 pounds (her highest weight). She felt well enough of herself to participate in a hospital-sponsored weight-loss program that required 3 months on a total liquid low-calorie diet. During the initial phase of this diet she was euphoric over her rapid weight loss. However, she once again became angry at me for not complimenting her and for not fully appreciating her effort to lose weight. On the other hand, she received many compliments from friends and co-workers over her improved physical appearance. Ironically (or expectedly), her parents did not commend her for her loss of weight (50 pounds). Her fantasy of beginning a romantic relationship with me when she reached 150 pounds reemerged, although with less intensity. Her sexual fantasies about me were predominantly images of being held, comforted, and understood. Making love to me, like eating, calmed and soothed her. The following is a representative description:

> You're soothing . . . you listen and everything's all right as long as you're here . . . I don't feel like eating when I'm with you . . . after I make love to my husband I fantasize lying next to you—I feel satisfied, comforted, and complete. I have an image of a baby with a bottle . . . it soothes all kinds of feelings—frustration, helplessness, anger, loneliness, boredom . . . it's more important than anything else.

She noted that when she had a "good" therapy session in which she felt understood and supported, she was able to leave without experiencing an impulse to eat. On the other hand, when she felt misunderstood or rejected by me, she experienced an intense desire to eat after the session. Satisfactory therapy sessions, similar to productive days at work, made her feel happy, excited, and enthusiastic. These feelings rarely evoked a compulsion to eat.

At the present time she weighs 225 pounds, which is almost exactly what she weighed at the beginning of treatment. Although her weight is the same, her feelings about herself are vastly different. She is considerably less self-deragatory about her physical appearance and places less emphasis on it. Her self-concept is better integrated without the polarity of a thin or fat self. She views herself as professionally competent, likeable, generous, and more tolerant of her own shortcomings as well as those of others. Her relationships with men are less anxiety-producing, and she occasionally permits herself the pleasure of a heterosexual fantasy without substituting a homosexual fantasy as a defensive maneuver. Her relationship with her husband has improved although she maintains that if she found someone more compatible and satisfying she could give up her compulsive eating entirely. This fantasy continues to include myself, although she has begun to entertain the possibility of termination again. The prospect of ending her therapeutic relationship with me still terrifies her, but she appears to have gained enough of a positive self-representation so that she can at least consider the possibility of sustaining herself without my continued availability for self-soothing.

DISCUSSION

I have presented this patient in order to illustrate the psychodynamics connected with compulsive eating, weight fluctuations, body image, and self-representation. I have also attempted to demonstrate the relationship of these dynamics to developmental phases and transference phenomena as they evolved during treatment. Keeping these issues in mind, I would like to briefly summarize each phase of treatment.

During the initial phase of treatment the patient's intense positive transference fueled her efforts to lose 60 pounds. One might say that this weight loss represented a "transference cure." However, she was unable to attain her goal of 150 pounds because of the near-panic generated by approaching the weight at which she fantasized seducing me. In addition, her weight loss did little to alter her self- and body image fundamentally. She continued to view herself as fat, inferior, unloveable, and sexually undesirable. It became evident that her compulsive eating temporarily neutralized a variety of feelings: anxiety, anger, sadness, emptiness, boredom, and despair. Moreover, her large body size enabled her to avoid sexual pleasure in fantasy as well as in reality. A polarized self-representation emerged in which she defined herself in terms of a thin or a fat self. Her inability to terminate when she neared her desired weight, as well as her rage at me for failing actively to dissuade her from terminating, set the stage for the next phase of therapy.

The second phase of treatment was characterized by continued weight fluctuations in association with oscillations of transference and self-image. She perceived me as alternately uncaring, insensitive, and critical, or as warm, supportive, and understanding. The negative components of her transference were related to longstanding feelings toward her mother whom she experienced as unloving, critical, and unattuned to her needs. Her father seemed to play a less prominent role transferentially; nonetheless, she found him (and myself) ineffectual, distant, and unwilling or unable to compensate for her mother's rejection. Fantasies, dreams, and associations further illuminated oedipal and preoedipal determinants of her hyperphagia. Overeating was a symbolic expression of her oedipal wishes as well as a defense against the anxiety and guilt they generated. Her unattractive body discouraged men from finding her sexually attractive, and indicated to other women that she presented a minimal competitive threat to them. The preoedipal origins of her compulsive eating were connected to a deeply frustrated desire for her mother's love, acceptance, and emotional responsiveness. Moreover, her overeating was, at times, a defiant, rageful act meant as a retaliation against her mother. Her sexual inhibitions and homosexual fantasies constituted a defense against the anxiety connected with her oedipal wishes, and simultaneously reflected her strong need for an approving, caring, intuitively responsive mother. By becoming pregnant, she not only acted out her oedipal wishes, but also tried to internalize deeply longed-for qualities from her mother (love, empathy) through incorporation of myself via a baby. She continued to struggle with her thin and fat-selves, vividly portrayed by the "cat dream" in which she rescued those parts of herself she valued and hoped to expand further.

During the third phase of treatment she took significant strides toward developing an integrated, positive self-representation. She was able to place less emphasis on her bodily self and the connotations of inferiority, ugliness, and unacceptability it held for her. Consequently, she felt less critical of her own body as well as the physical appearance of other obese individuals. She gradually strengthened those parts of herself she valued: intellectual curiosity, spontaneity, humor, generosity, assertiveness, and the ability to empathize. Her ambivalent transference evolved into a more realistically based perception of myself, along with feeling respected and accepted by me. Nevertheless, she continues to harbor a fantasy of my ultimately falling in love with her, thus achieving an oedipal triumph and a reunion with an idealized mother. It has become more clearly evident that her compulsive eating is a "self-soothing" mechanism aimed at the neutralization of dysphoric states. Food remains a transitional object (as I do myself) providing her with emotional gratification and security. However, pleasurable moods connected with being understood or feeling competent and effective do not trigger hyperphagia. In conjunction with the development of a more cohesive, positive self-image, she has been able to lose a significant amount of weight. Termination also seems a more likely possibility now that she has achieved a reasonably stable internalized sense of being understood and valued.

I believe that resistance and countertransference issues encountered during her treatment are worthy of comment. Throughout therapy she has periodically attempted to coerce me into taking an active role in helping her to lose weight (e.g., monitoring her weight, etc.). If I were her internist I would have gladly done so. However, as her analyst, I have tried to steer a "neutral" course on this matter because I have wanted to avoid the appearance of favoring her thin self over her fat self. To have done so would have placed me in the position of rejecting or devaluing a part of herself, however, unacceptable to her. In addition, I would have colluded with her magical, irrational expectations associated with weight loss. However, maintaining a "neutral" attitude on this matter has frequently subjected me to charges of being uncaring or indifferent. These criticisms have reinforced a frequent sense of never quite giving enough of myself to her. Occasionally, I have reacted defensively by becoming oversolicitous, withholding, or annoyed. In general, I have tried to be empathic without intervening, as far as dieting and weight loss are concerned. I believe that my attempt to accept unqualifiedly both her thin and fat selves has served a self-object function that she has successfully internalized. Moreover, I believe that understanding and empathizing with her emotional deprivations rather than focussing exclusively on their irrational aspects, has enabled her gradually to accept rather than condemn her entire self. Similar to other patients suffering from psychophysiological disorders or chronic physical illness, I have repeatedly told her that she is struggling with biological forces that may be beyond her control and that place limitations on the ultimate weight she might attain. At the risk of appearing pessimistic, I believe that this approach has helped somewhat to lessen her conscious sense of guilt over not losing enough weight. In part, I have considered her preoccupation with her weight and physical appearance as forms of resistance that have had to be explored patiently in order to comprehend and interpret their unconscious sources. On the other hand, I have grown to appreciate how exquisitely painful it has been for her to possess a body that others have overtly or covertly devalued, rejected, or ridiculed. As a result, I have come to admire her courage in continuing to effect internal changes, despite a relatively refractory external appearance. As far as her repeated attempts to terminate are concerned, I have basically viewed them as tests of my emotional availability and commitment to help her. Although her lengthy treatment might be viewed as a continuing effort on her part to hold me as a transitional object, I believe that she has also required that amount of time to internalize and consolidate my maternally-soothing qualities successfully.

The observations I have made from this single case study appear to support the conclusions of the Academy study in regard to the treatment of obesity. Namely, treatment improves self- and body image, while psychodynamic issues are clearly associated with hyperphagia and weight changes. In the Academy study, psychodynamic issues connected with emotional gratification and deprivation were predominant (Glucksman et al., 1978). For this patient, a profoundly disturbed relationship with her mother seemed to be the crucial factor in her failure to develop a well-internalized sense of self capable of effective self-soothing. Nevertheless, it is difficult, if not impossible to ascribe her obesity to disturbances in her early feeding experiences. There is insufficient data either from anamnesis or direct observations to conclude that her oral phase of development was poorly negotiated. We can only infer from her memories, fantasies, and dreams that she experienced a qualitatively deficient amount of maternal nurturing during the oral phase. The clinical material clearly demonstrates that her abnormal eating pattern and impaired self-image are etiologically connected to conflicts at the preoedipal, oedipal, and postoedipal developmental stages. In view of this, her compulsive eating and self-pathology can be considered the sequelae of a long-standing, severely disturbed total relationship with her mother (and to a lesser extent her father) that adversely affected each phase of development. Perhaps, only long-term prospective studies of maternal–infant interaction (including feeding) will provide us with the necessary data in order to understand more fully the relationship between inadequate maternal care-giving during the initial months of life and the development of obesity.

Although her weight has fluctuated within a range of nearly 100 pounds over the course of treatment, she has had virtually no net loss of weight. The Academy study demonstrated significant net losses of weight after 4 years of treatment; this patient has been in treatment for a considerably longer duration. Taking into consideration the undeniable relationship between compulsive eating, weight gain, weight loss, and psychodynamic issues, what other factors might have contributed to her inability to maintain a significantly lower weight? Obviously, hereditary, metabolic, morphologic, and neurochemical influences must be taken into account. Recent studies suggest the presence of a significant genetic component to obesity. Stunkard et al. (1986) observed a strong relationship between the weights of adoptees and the body-mass index of their biological parents. Conversely, there was no correlation between the weights of adoptees and the body-mass index of their adoptive parents. This genetic influence was not confined to the obesity weight class alone, but was displayed across the entire range of body fatness — from very thin to very fat. On the basis of this as well as other studies (Borjeson, 1976) there appears to be little doubt that genetic factors play an important role in the predisposition to obesity. Two studies recently published demonstrate that reduced energy expenditure is an important factor contributing to obesity among infants born to overweight mothers and also among certain southwestern American Indian families (Ravussin et al., 1988; Roberts et al., 1988). These findings indicate a genetic influence that predisposes certain individuals and families to lower rates of energy expenditure and a higher risk of becoming obese. There is also evidence that abnormalities of fat cell morphology (hypertrophy and hyperplasia) in children and adults who become obese may play a role in determining the extent to which permanent weight loss is possible (Hirsch and Knittle, 1970). Because of these genetic, metabolic and morphologic factors, it may be extremely difficult for obese individuals (including the patient I have presented) to maintain a significantly lowered body weight over a prolonged period of time, effective psychotherapy notwithstanding.

Some obese individuals seem to crave carbohydrate-rich foods while others do not. Studies have shown that obese carbohydrate-cravers report feeling less depressed, calmer, and more relaxed following the ingestion of carbohydrate-rich meals (Lieberman et al., 1986; Wurtman and Wurtman, 1986). Changes in serotonergic neurotransmission may be partially responsible for the affective change following carbohydrate consumption. Carbohydrate ingestion raises brain tryptophan levels, thereby accelerating the synthesis and release of serotonin. The latter is intimately involved in mood alteration and exerts antidepressant effects. Therefore, certain obese individuals, similar to the drug addicts described by Khantzian (1985), may select carbohydrate-rich foods in order to self-medicate when they experience painful feelings, particularly those in the depressive spectrum. Many obese patients, including the one I have discussed, often report sad, empty, yearning, lonely feelings. Although these feelings are often linked to preoedipal dynamics, (e.g., inadequate maternal care-giving), they may be soothed and diminished temporarily through the ingestion of foods high in carbohydrate content. The addictive-like eating patterns of this group of obese individuals may be partially explained on the basis of the neurochemical sequence activated by carbohydrate ingestion.

In summary, although therapy can be effective in promoting positive changes in self and body-image for obese patients, it may not be as effective in bringing about a permanently lowered body weight. The Academy study as well as my case illustration clearly document a relationship between compulsive eating, weight fluctuations, emotions, body image, self-representation, and specific psychodynamic issues. The latter appear to be the product of disturbances throughout childhood and adolescent development, particularly in the area of mother–child interaction. Inappropriate or deficient maternal emotional attunement and responsivity seem to play an especially crucial role. However, there is insufficient data to implicate the feeding process during the oral phase of development as a primary etiological factor. Although hyperphagia and weight fluctuations definitely articulate with psychodynamic processes, there are underlying genetic, metabolic, morphologic, and neurochemical phenomena that exert a profound influence on body weight over an extended period of time. Similar to other psychophysiological disorders, obesity appears to be the final common pathway resulting from a complex interaction between critical developmental experiences and genetically determined biological processes.

References

Alexander, F. (1934), The influence of psychological factors upon gastrointestinal disturbances, *Psychoanal. Quart., 3*, 501–539.

Borjeson, M. (1976), The aetiology of obesity in children: A study of 101 twin pairs, *Acta Pediat. Scand., 65*, 279–287.

Bruch, H. (1957), *The Importance of Overweight*, W. W. Norton, New York.

Bruch, H. (1961), Conceptual confusion in eating disorders, *J. Nerv. Ment. Dis., 133*, 46–54.

Bychowski, G. (1950), On neurotic obesity, *Psychoanal. Rev., 37*, 301–319.

Castelnuovo-Tedesco, P., and Reiser, L. W. (1988), Compulsive eating: Obesity and related phenomena, panel report, *J. Am. Psychoanal. Assoc., 36*, 163–171.

Freud, A. (1972), The psychoanalytic study of infantile feeding disorders, in S. Harrison and J. McDermitt (Eds.), *Childhood Psychopathology*, International Universities Press, New York.

Freud, S. (1905), Three essays on the theory of sexuality, *Standard Edition*, Hogarth Press, London, 1953, Vol. 7, pp. 179–184.

Glucksman, M. L. (1968), The response of obese patients to weight reduction: A clinical evaluation of behavior, *Psychosom. Med., 30*, 1–11.

Glucksman, M. L. (1972), Psychiatric observations on obesity, *Adv. Psychosom. Med., 7*, 194–216.

Glucksman, M. L., and Hirsch, J. (1969), The response of obese patients to weight reduction: III. The perception of body size, *Psychosom. Med., 31*, 1–7.

Glucksman, M. L., Rand, C. S. W., and Stunkard, A. J. (1978), Psychodynamics of obesity, *J. Am. Acad. Psychoanal., 6*, 103–115.

Goodsitt, A. (1983), Self-regulatory disturbances in eating disorders, *Int. J. Eating Disorders, 2*, 51–60.

Hamburger, W. W. (1951), Emotional aspects of obesity, *Med. Clin. N. Amer., 35*, 483–499.

Hirsch, J., and Knittle, J. L. (1970), Cellularity of obese and non-obese human adipose tissue, *Fed. Proc., 29*, 1516–1521.

Kaplan, H. I., and Kaplan, H. S. (1957), The psychosomatic concept of obesity, *J. Nerv. Ment. Dis., 125*, 181–201.

Khantzian, E. J. (1985), The self-medication hypothesis of addictive disorders: Focus on heroin and cocaine dependence, *Am. J. Psychiatry, 142*, 1259–1264.

Kohut, H. (1971), *The Analysis of the Self*, International Universities Press, New York.

Kohut, H. (1977), *The Restoration of the Self*, International Universities Press, New York.

Levy, D. (1934), Primary Affect Hunger, *Am. J. Psychiatry, 94*, 643–652.

Lieberman, H. R., Wurtman, J. J., and Chew, B. (1986), Changes in mood after carbohydrate consumption among obese individuals, *Am. J. Clin. Nutr., 44*, 772–778.

Mahler, M. S., Pine, F., and Bergman, A. (1975), *The Psychological Birth of the Human Infant*, Basic Books, New York.

Modell, A. (1976), The "holding environment" and the therapeutic action of psychoanalysis, *J. Am. Psychoanal. Assoc., 24*, 285–307.

Ornstein, A. (1981), Self-pathology in childhood: Developmental and clinical considerations, *Psychiatric Clinics of North America, 4*, 435–453.

Rand, C. S. W., and Stunkard, A. J. (1977), Psychoanalysis and obesity, *J. Am. Acad. Psychoanal., 5*, 459–497.

Rand, C. S. W., and Stunkard, A. J. (1978), Obesity and psychoanalysis, *Am. J. Psychiatry, 135*, 547–551.

Rand, C. S. W., and Stunkard, A. J. (1983), Obesity and psychoanalysis: Treatment and four-year follow-up, *Am. J. Psychiatry, 140*, 1140–1144.

Rascovsky, A., DeRascovsky, M. W., and Schlossberg, T. (1950), *Int. J. Psycho-Anal., 31*, 144–149.

Ravussin, E., Lillioja, S., Knowler, W. C., Christin, L., Freymond, D., Abbott, W. G. H., Boyce, V., Howard, B. V., and Bogardus, C. (1988), Reduced rate of energy expenditure as a risk factor for body-weight gain, *N. Eng. J. Med., 318*, 467–472.

Raynes, E. (1987), The effects of developmental relationships on eating behavior in adult women, Ph.D. dissertation, Yeshiva Univ., New York.

Roberts, S. B., Savage, J., Coward, W. A., Chew, B., and Lucas, A. (1988), Energy expenditure and intake in infants born to lean and overweight mothers, *N. Eng. J. Med., 318*, 461–466.

Slochower, J. A. (1983), *Excessive Eating: The Role of Emotions and Environment*, Human Sciences Press, New York.

Spitz, R. (1965), *First Year of Life*, International Universities Press, New York.

Stunkard, A. J., and Koch, C. (1964), The interpretation of gastric motility: I. Apparent bias in the reports of hunger by obese persons, *Arch. Gen. Psychiatry, 11*, 74–82.

Stunkard, A. J., Sorensen, T. I. A., Hanis, C., Teasdale, T. W., Chakraborty, R., Schull, W. J., and Schulsinger, F. (1986), An adoption study of human obesity, *N. Eng. J. Med., 314*, 193–198.

Tolpin, M. (1971), On the beginnings of a cohesive self, *Psychoanal. Study Child, 26*, 316–352.

Winnicott, D. W. (1953), *Transitional Objects and Transitional Phenomena, Int. J. Psycho-Anal., 34*, 89–97.

Winnicott, D. W. (1965), *The Maturational Processes and the Facilitating Environment*, International Universities Press, Madison, CT.

Winnicott, D. W. (1971), *Playing and Reality*, Basic Books, New York.

Wurtman, R. J., and Wurtman, J. J. (1986), Carbohydrate craving, obesity and brain serotonin, *Appetite, 7*, 99–103.

27 Hospital Avenue
Danbury, CT 06810